BEYOND MEDICINE

A volume in the series
THE CULTURE AND POLITICS OF HEALTH CARE WORK

Edited by Suzanne Gordon and Sioban Nelson

For a list of books in the series, visit our website at cornellpress.cornell.edu.

BEYOND MEDICINE

*Why European Social Democracies
Enjoy Better Health Outcomes
Than the United States*

PAUL V. DUTTON

ILR PRESS
AN IMPRINT OF
CORNELL UNIVERSITY PRESS
ITHACA AND LONDON

First published 2021 by Cornell University Press

Library of Congress Cataloging-in-Publication Data

Names: Dutton, Paul V., author.
Title: Beyond medicine : why European social democracies enjoy better health outcomes than the United States / Paul V. Dutton.
Description: Ithaca [New York] : Cornell University Press, 2021. | Series: The culture and politics of health care work | Includes bibliographical references and index.
Identifiers: LCCN 2020025549 (print) | LCCN 2020025550 (ebook) | ISBN 9781501754555 (hardcover) | ISBN 9781501754562 (paperback) | ISBN 9781501754586 (pdf) | ISBN 9781501754579 (epub)
Subjects: LCSH: Health—Social aspects—United States. | Health—Social aspects—Europe, Western. | Health—Political aspects—United States. | Health—Political aspects—Europe, Western. | Medical care—United States—History. | Medical care—Europe, Western—History. | Well-being—United States. | Well-being—Europe, Western.
Classification: LCC RA418.3.U6 D87 2021 (print) | LCC RA418.3.U6 (ebook) | DDC 362.1—dc23
LC record available at https://lccn.loc.gov/2020025549
LC ebook record available at https://lccn.loc.gov/2020025550

To Allan Mitchell,
teacher, mentor, friend

The idea of social democracy is now used to describe a society the economy of which is predominantly capitalist, but where the state acts to regulate the economy in the general interest, provides welfare services outside of it and attempts to alter the distribution of income and wealth in the name of social justice.

—*Routledge Encyclopedia of Philosophy*

CONTENTS

PREFACE

This book owes its origins to my experience of founding and directing an interdisciplinary health policy research institute at Northern Arizona University between 2008 and 2015. The institute brought together anthropologists, biologists, health scientists, hospital administrators, insurance executives, medical faculty, physicians, political scientists, psychologists, state legislators, public health officials, social workers, and many others. Amazingly, I never had to recruit any of them. Once word got out that we were working across disciplinary boundaries, dozens of talented people called, wanting to be involved. Every one of them was special. Each intuitively understood that no matter how great their individual achievements, large-scale solutions would require collaboration with others from across the health system—that health encompasses all dimensions of life and is therefore inescapably interdisciplinary. And that because of our incessant efforts to partition expertise into ever-more specialized fields we are losing sight of the big picture that is imperative to wise policy making.

As the director I had the privilege of participating in many institute projects and events. Two of them were especially formative to this book's emphasis on the social determinants of health and the potential for state action to improve them. In 2012, the public health researchers Priscilla Sanderson and Nicky Teufel-Shone won a large, multiyear grant from the National Institutes of Health to create the Center for American Indian Resilience (CAIR). Priscilla asked me to chair the executive advisory board, a group of eminent Native American leaders and health experts. Never before in my life has it been clearer to me that I should listen and that I should talk only when necessary. Native American leaders understand like no one else that health is about community. Unlike some of my other institute meetings where physicians were present, Navajo, Hopi or Tohono O'odham doctors never arrogated for themselves an outsized role in the struggle against serious health conditions. They spoke with expertise about medical matters yet yielded to others on the equal importance of poverty, racism, and the absence of opportunity. I came away from every CAIR board meeting with a deeper appreciation of the social determinants of health and a resolve to bring those understandings to my own research.

The institute also held health policy roundtables for the stakeholders of Arizona's health system. We modeled these annual events on the Aspen Institute Seminar. Participants agreed in advance to ground rules that included confidentiality, empathetic listening, and the objective of finding common ground. By far, the deepest policy division of the time was whether Arizona should expand its Medicaid program under the 2010 Affordable Care Act. With a Republican governor and Republican majorities in control of both houses of the state legislature it seemed unlikely that Arizona would go along with Obamacare. Our roundtables included the state's Medicaid director and the governor's health policy advisor. Also in attendance were Democratic and Republican state legislators, rural hospital CEOs, insurance executives, large hospital CMOs, physicians, researchers, county health directors, and others; we capped attendance at thirty-two. In facilitating the roundtables, I was surprised to learn that today's health politics resemble those of the nineteenth and early twentieth centuries. Ideological and partisan divides are important, but they are joined by many other concerns. In June 2013, Arizona governor Jan Brewer worked with Democratic lawmakers and a few moderate Republicans to defeat her own party's legislative majorities to expand Arizona

Medicaid under the Affordable Care Act. Her action extended health coverage to over three hundred thousand low-income workers and their children. When diverse stakeholders unite, they can influence state power in surprising ways. The following history recounts many such instances in hopes of illuminating the potential for future state action to improve the opportunity for all to live healthy lives.

Paul V. Dutton
Tucson, Arizona

Acknowledgments

Historians rely on the traces left behind by others. We interpret their actions by connecting them with other people, patterns, and possibilities in order to make sense of the past. Yet this task becomes more difficult the closer we approach the present. We lack too much of the perspective that only the passage of time can provide. For this reason, I owe a tremendous debt to my colleagues in economics, medical sociology, epidemiology, and the health sciences. Their accomplishments made it possible for me to navigate the treacherous straits of the recent past and to emerge into the light of present day. Specialists of all kinds will, no doubt, find omissions in my analysis. This is only natural. I only ask that they bear in mind the breadth of the comparative project at hand. I sometimes had to simplify my language and to condense detail to reach as broad an audience as possible.

Several individuals gave gifts of time and expertise. My editor at Cornell University Press, Suzanne Gordon, supported the project from the beginning, and her professional eye never faltered; she provided constructive criticism right up to the end. Over a long Parisian lunch, Elodie

Richard listened carefully as I poured out my confusion over how to organize the unwieldy past of European and American health institutions and outcomes. Then she calmly suggested the comparative approach that follows. I hope I have done justice to her idea. My friend Ray Michalowski provided incisive observations and advice on early drafts. Paul-André Rosenthal loaned me his lectern for a day at Sciences Po, Romain Huret did the same at the École des Hautes Études en Sciences Sociales, and Bruno Valat invited me to address his research working group at the Université de Toulouse-Mirail. I am grateful for these opportunities to share my ideas with advanced graduate students and faculty; they contributed immeasurably to this book.

Many others provided precious encouragement, if only to suggest yet another book to read or to reassure me that what I was doing would eventually bear fruit. These include Shipra Bansal, Ellen Boucher, Doug Campos-Outcalt, Christophe Capuano, Mark Carroll, Bob England, Tom Finger, John Haeger, Lisa Hardy, Eric Henley, Eileen Kline, Cheryl Koos, Amelia Lyon, Julia Lynch, Julia Moses, Michelle Parsons, Lance Price, Andy Saal, Fred Solop, Priscilla Sanderson, Dana Simmons, Steve Sokol, Robert Trotter, Greg Vigdor, Neil Warrence, and Bill Wiist. They contributed more to the project than they know.

This book could not have been completed without financial and institutional support. Grants from the American Philosophical Society, the Fulbright Program, and the Office of the Associate Provost for Research and Graduate Studies at Northern Arizona University made possible extended research sojourns in the United States and Europe. In addition, I would like to extend my appreciation to the chair of the history department at Northern Arizona University, Derek Heng, for shielding my research from administrative and bureaucratic interruptions, a thankless but indispensable role of a university department chair. Lastly, I owe the greatest thanks to my family. To Linden for her help on finding a title, to Diana who rescued me from frustration with the illustrations, and to Finley for his brutally honest take on everything. And to my best friend and wife, Shelby, whose insights as a health care provider lent a much-needed dose of firsthand knowledge to my historical analysis. Her confidence and commitment sustained me throughout the project.

BEYOND MEDICINE

INTRODUCTION

Relative Decline Is Decline All the Same

We have a health care system in the United States which is not very
well set up to save lives or to keep us healthy but which does make a
lot of people very rich as it's terribly expensive.

—ANGUS DEATON, INTERVIEW WITH FREAKONOMICS RADIO

The superstar investor Warren Buffett once pointed out that "it's only
when the tide goes out that you learn who's been swimming naked."[1]
The COVID-19 pandemic was just such a tide. In a few weeks it brutally
exposed the nakedness of Americans who have been swimming in an
ocean teeming with threats to their health—biological, social, and
economic—for many decades. This book argues that a nation's health system must be constructed in order to protect people's health from many
culprits, such as infectious disease and lack of medical care, but also social
factors like financial insecurity, housing shortages, and racial discrimination, all of which influence one's opportunity to live a healthy life. I argue
that we should reconceive the boundaries of our health system well beyond medicine and that health must be understood in historical terms.
Only by analyzing how health systems have performed under the duress of
the great historic challenges of the modern era, namely industrialization,
urbanization, the world wars, and the Great Depression, can we render

judgements on how well they will fare against present challenges, such as globalization, climate change, and pandemics.

What follows is a comparative history of the US health system, measuring it against three European social democracies: France, Germany, and Sweden. As social democracies, these nations possess predominantly capitalist economies, but their governments regulate those economies in the general interest. They ensure high-quality universal social safety nets and seek a reasonable balance in the distribution of wealth and income, not only in the name of social justice but also because financial security is an important determinant in the health of their people.[2]

The COVID-19 pandemic demonstrated the strengths of social democratic health systems while simultaneously exposing analogous weaknesses in the United States. For example, when COVID-19 first appeared in Europe and the United States in early 2020, French, German, and Swedish workers could rely on substantial dedicated paid sick leave to slow the rate of infection. In contrast, 28 percent of American workers possess no dedicated paid sick leave, and many of these occupy low-wage positions in food service and retail commerce; they were on average more vulnerable to infection and more likely to infect others.[3] Some of these workers inevitably had to choose between paying rent or going to work when they felt ill. By April 2020, when the pandemic had emerged as the most acute infectious disease crisis in living memory, analysts predicted that some 9.2 million US workers would lose their employer-provided health insurance due to layoffs caused by the slowing of economic activity.[4] French, German, and Swedish workers faced no such absurdity, their nations having decades ago achieved universal health coverage that is not dependent on employment status. In another failing of the US health system, many American workers who remained employed in essential services found themselves without sufficient workplace protections from infection, circumstances that were belatedly rectified by employers but only after the firing of a worker who led others in protest.[5] In contrast, when Amazon France failed to quickly ensure safe working conditions, a high court sided with the workers' union, ordering Amazon to provide paid furloughs to the affected employees until occupational safety conditions had been ameliorated.[6]

Meanwhile, the US health care system—by far the most expensive in the world—demonstrated shallow preparedness in the face of a long-predicted epidemic of infectious respiratory disease.[7] Shortages of personal protective equipment, ventilators, diagnostic and antibody test kits, and even the swabs required to use the test kits were all in short supply.[8] To be sure, German hospitals were in crisis mode, calling in medical students to fill key provider roles, and personal protective equipment was in short supply, but they never lacked ventilators or intensive-care treatment beds.[9] Indeed, the German case fatality rate emerged as among the lowest in the world because early in the crisis the nation rapidly increased its production of high-quality test kits. Pervasive diagnostic testing and contact tracing permitted health authorities to control local outbreaks.[10] Meanwhile, in the United States, widespread transmission of the virus went undetected, causing a loss of valuable time during which self-isolation and quarantines would have significantly reduced the rate of infection and deaths. By April, Germany, with 82,000,000 inhabitants, was conducting 120,000 COVID-19 antibody tests per day, including random sampling across the nation, providing valuable epidemiological data. At that point in the pandemic, US testing was rising rapidly but still woefully short, at 146,000 tests per day in a nation of 330,000,000 inhabitants.[11] Then, as political pressure built to lift shelter-in-place orders and to reopen businesses in May, President Donald Trump, who had earlier insisted on absolute federal control of the crisis, abruptly relinquished federal responsibility. He directed governors to manage their own testing and to decide their own reopening schedules, even though their capability to do so varied widely across the nation.[12]

Sweden never substantially closed down its economy, not due to zigzagging national policies but because of a conscious decision to adopt a markedly different approach to COVID-19. Under the advice of Sweden's Public Health Agency, the government issued social distancing directives, banned gatherings greater than eighty people, and closed high schools and colleges. But preschools and elementary schools remained open, restaurants, cafes, and stores continued to operate, and about half of the labor force who could work from home were asked to do so. The Public Health Agency, mindful that shutting down the economy had negative health effects of its own, sought to attenuate rather than entirely suppress infection rates, especially among the young whose vulnerability to the worst effects of the disease were statistically quite low. Sweden's strategy aimed to preserve acute-care treatment capacity while building herd immunity by metering the transmission of the virus through the population. Overall, Sweden's case fatality rates have proven comparable to other European nations, though older Swedes, especially those living in group retirement homes, experienced higher death rates than the elderly in neighboring Scandinavian countries who sheltered in place and enacted more severe economic shutdowns.[13]

A comprehensive assessment of health system performance and outcomes during the COVID-19 pandemic must await future historians. However, during the initial months, France, Germany, and Sweden demonstrated greater resilience than the United States across a broad range of societal responses. French workers could protect themselves from viral infection because unions possess significant power over occupational health conditions; the nation's commercial and retail supply chains are also less beholden to a single online retailer. The German government could leapfrog unreliable market incentives to ensure a massive increase in antibody test kits because the nation's pharmaceutical expertise has long been protected alongside the state's ability to deploy it in an emergency. The Swedish Public Health Agency's seemingly radical plan to obtain herd immunity was only possible because the nation already possessed universal health care, integrated health and social service providers, and widespread public confidence in both. Moreover, France, Germany, and Sweden possess healthier populations, a fundamental element of resilience when infectious disease strikes.

The majority of adults hospitalized with COVID-19 in the United States have underlying medical conditions. Indeed, during March 2020, nearly half (49.7 percent) suffered from hypertension, 48.3 percent were obese, 38.6 percent had chronic lung disease, 28.3 percent suffered from diabetes mellitus, and 27.8 percent had cardiovascular disease. Age also emerged as a significant risk. Some three-quarters of those hospitalized were over forty-nine years old.[14] The US population is younger than Europe's, but both are growing older at a steady clip. By 2050, 22 percent of Americans and 27 percent of Europeans will be over age sixty-four.[15] However, despite their tandem aging trends, Americans exhibit much higher rates of disease prevalence than Europeans among those age fifty and older: 17.1 percent higher for hypertension, 10.4 percent higher for heart disease, 6.8 percent higher for cancer, and 5.5 percent higher for diabetes.[16] Unfortunately, in contrast to the aging trends whereby the US and European populations are both growing older, Americans are growing sicker than their European counterparts with each passing year.[17] If we are to understand this trend and identify how it might be arrested, the US health system performance must be examined historically and in comparison to other nations. The airwaves, op-ed pages, and social media are full of earnest (and not-so-earnest) arguments about how the United States might improve. But we should start by considering the actual health of Americans—that is, our population *health outcomes*, how they compare to similar-income nations, why they are relatively poor, and what we might do in order to improve them.

Health outcomes fall into two broad categories: *mortality* and *health-related quality of life*. Mortality refers to life expectancy at birth. For example, Americans' life expectancy is 78.6 years; French life expectancy is 82.3. Mortality may also be reported concerning a specific condition or event to which death is attributed, such as infant mortality, maternal mortality, motor-vehicle accidents, cancer, or ischemic heart disease. All are reported in proportion to population size. For example, the German infant mortality rate is 3.2 per one thousand live births; the American infant mortality rate is 5.8 per one thousand live births. In contrast to mortality, health-related quality of life outcomes capture health status and are measured in functional terms drawn from clinical data and surveys. For example, 43 percent of Americans over age sixty-five are classified as "high need." They suffer from multiple chronic conditions and a diminished capacity to perform the activities of daily living. Only 28 percent of Swedes over age sixty-five are deemed high need.[18]

In addition to describing the average health of a nation, health outcomes also provide crucial information about the distribution of health among population subgroups according to race, ethnicity, socioeconomic class, gender, sexual orientation, and other criteria. These data are essential to the identification of health inequities and the formulation of policies to rectify them. US maternal mortality is a particularly distressing example. In contrast to similar-income nations, the US rate has been rising, not falling, in recent decades. In 1987, seven out of every 100,000 pregnant American women died of child-birth-related causes. By 2018, maternal mortality had risen to 26.4 per 100,000. African American women of all socioeconomic backgrounds are now more than three times as likely to die during pregnancy or childbirth-related causes than non-Hispanic white women.[19] If a defective American-made jetliner crashed every year, killing eight hundred American mothers—the current maternal

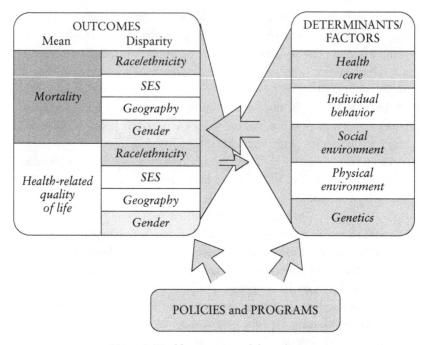

Figure 1. Health outcomes and determinants.

Source: "What Are Population Health Outcomes?," *Improving Population Health*, 2020, https://www.improvingpopulationhealth.org/blog/what-are-population-health-outcomes.html.

death toll—while a European airplane operated without incident we would demand to know why.[20] But rarely does one hear something like, "Many European nations have cut their maternal mortality rate in half since 1990, and it's now less than a third the US rate, and they spend a lot less on health care than we do—perhaps they have found some solutions we should consider."[21]

Medical Care and the Social Determinants of Health

Even when the health outcomes of Americans are compared to other nations, the emphasis rarely departs from the subject of medical treatment, pharmaceuticals, and health insurance. The prescriptions are familiar: create Medicare for All, regulate drug prices, deregulate health insurance companies, recognize access to health care as a right, develop personalized medicine—the list could go on. Indeed, since the 1910s Americans have argued about whether and how to implement a system of universal health care. Unfortunately, these recurring political debates have distracted us from the social determinants of health, which are more influential over health outcomes than medical care. The sociologist Kathryn Strother Ratcliff puts it well. Social determinants, she says, are "the conditions of life people are exposed to because of the way their society is built—how we live, how we work, how we move from place to place, and what we eat and drink."[22] Such conditions include household financial security, employment stability and stress, access to preventive and curative medical services, the availability of clean water and healthful food, the safety and healthfulness of housing, neighborhoods, and transportation. Epidemiological studies have distinguished the broad social determinants of health from the effects of individual traits and the health care system.[23] The results of two of the most important of these studies are illustrated below. We see that individual biology, genetic endowment, and lifestyle choices such as smoking and diet are all major factors. But the physical, social, and economic environments constitute the more dominant influences over our health.[24] This is not to say that social and physical factors determine the health of any one individual. Rather, these studies indicate what causes the average health of populations as well as the health inequities between groups within those populations. As the epidemiologists Michael Marmot and Jessica Allen put it, "so close is the link between social conditions and health, that the magnitude of health inequalities is an indicator of the impact of social and economic inequalities on people's lives."[25] Health status has thus become a reliable gauge by which we can observe the rapid rise in wealth and income inequality.

Still, in the United States, a great illusion persists that better medicine is responsible for the dramatic progress in life expectancy and health outcomes over the last century. Between 1750 and 1950 life expectancy increased more than in all of previous history. But most improvements occurred prior to and independently of discoveries in germ theory or advances in preventive and curative medicine. Even the dazzling breakthroughs of the mid-twentieth century, including vaccines, pharmaceutical therapies, surgery, and diagnostic imaging account for only between 10 and 20 percent of improved health in the United States and other

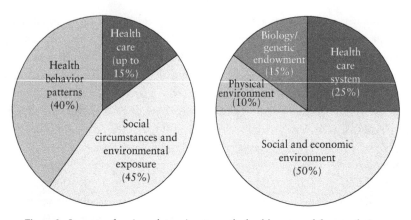

Figure 2. Impacts of various determinants on the health status of the population.

Source: Canadian Institute of Advanced Research, Health Canada, Population and Public Health Branch, cited in Daria Kuznetsova, *Healthy Places: Councils Leading on Public Health* (London: New Local Government Network, 2012), http://www.nlgn.org.uk/public/ 2012/healthy-places-councils-leading-on-public-health; J. M. McGinnis et al., "The Case for More Active Policy Attention to Health Promotion," *Health Affairs* 21, no. 2 (March/April 2002): 78–93, https://doi.org/10.1377/hlthaff.21.2.78.

developed nations. Put differently, better medicine can claim credit for only about five years of the thirty-year increase in US life expectancy over the course of the twentieth century.[26]

In large measure, Americans' overestimation of medical care's importance is due to what political economist Robert Crawford calls *healthism*. Healthism is a preoccupation with the individual in understanding the causes of sickness and ill-being. It locates the primary causes of disease in deficient individual bodies and ignores the predominant influences of the social and physical environments. It insists that the individual must cope with objectively unhealthy circumstances, whether substandard housing, unstable employment, or financial insecurity. By exaggerating the individual's responsibility, healthism shields harmful social institutions and practices from reform even though they are the greater causes of ill health.[27] Let us take the example of a community whose children are constantly sick due to a shortage of quality, affordable childcare. The childcare centers available to modest-income families must rely on very few staff and accept too many children for their facilities, contributing to the spread of communicable disease. Moreover, the overburdened childcare providers possess little time to coordinate their operations with local public health authorities. According to healthism, the parents and the children themselves are to blame for the serial sicknesses. The institutional failure that lies behind the children's poor health is invisible because social institutions are not individual bodies and cannot harbor or cause disease. Social circumstances must be accepted as unfortunate, unalterable circumstances with which the parents must cope.

Healthism is also implicated in the medicalization of our perception of health. Indeed, the two have been mutually reinforcing throughout the development of modern medicine. Prior to the eighteenth century, medical students were required to memorize medical theories that dated from Greek and Roman times, namely the writings of Hippocrates and Galen. Then, beginning in the 1760s, professors at the Paris School of Medicine replaced the rote memorization of ancient texts with new, empirical methods that were also propelling advancements in other sciences. They taught their students through experimental surgery, dissection, and autopsy. They commanded students: *"Peu lire, beaucoup voir!"* ("Read less, see more!") The Paris School built surgical amphitheaters (the term "surgical amphitheater" remains in use on hospital wards today), where students could observe the latest medical expertise. The new techniques revealed human anatomy and physiology like never before. They laid the foundation for nineteenth-century breakthroughs in germ theory, which also relied on experimentation and observation, aided by advancements in microscopy, chemistry, and biology. Doctors benefited greatly from these developments. Now able to comprehend the basic function of bodily organs and to see previously invisible pathogens, physicians vastly improved their diagnosis and therapy. Life-saving vaccines and antiseptics soon followed, helped by better anesthesia, permitting surgery inside the large body cavities that had previously been off limits. From these breakthroughs was born the modern medicine that we know today.

With ever greater knowledge and healing capabilities, physicians captured more prestige and political power. Doctors now understood the human body in previously unimagined ways and could achieve unprecedented feats of individual healing. Soon they asserted the right to name and define not only disease but health itself. And they did so, not surprisingly, through physicians' eyes. Thus empowered, it should come as little surprise that many physicians came to believe that ill health was located primarily within individual bodies and could only be repaired at the hands of a physician. The more effective the doctors became at individual healing, the more individuals turned to doctors in pursuit of health, the greater the influence of healthism. The medicalization of health was complete.[28]

Yet despite massive expenditures to conquer ill health through medicalization, American health outcomes have stalled compared to similar-income nations in Europe. The United States annually spends $3.6 trillion or 17.8 percent of its gross domestic product (GDP) on health care or $10,224 per person annually; the average spending of other high-income nations is 11.5 percent of GDP or $5,280 dollars per person annually.[29] Still, access to medical care for millions of Americans remains uncertain, and the cost of insurance and prescription drugs continues to rise at rates above general inflation. Moreover, the intensive practice of powerful medicine without proper coordination has meant that medical errors are so common in the United States that medical care itself is the third leading cause of death after heart disease and cancer.[30] Since people know about the expense and lack of access, if not the dangers, polls have long indicated that most Americans believe their health care system needs rebuilding.[31] But major reform attempts have occurred less than once per decade since 1910, and less than half of these have succeeded.

Only the boldest political leaders have ventured into health care reform, fearful of powerful interest groups, especially specialty physician groups, insurers, pharmaceutical firms, and health care corporations. Most American leaders have preferred to practice a *politics of disease* rather than a *politics of health*. Initiatives that focus on specific diseases and conditions, such as polio, renal failure, cancers of all kinds, HIV-AIDS, and autism have been politically safer.[32] Much of the health care industry and philanthropic foundations are similarly disposed toward the politics (and economics) of disease rather than health. There are now more ribbon colors than there are months of the year. New disease campaigns, sometimes promoted by pharmaceutical firms that stand to gain, must either share colors or create new fads. Meanwhile, the social and physical determinants of health, whose amelioration would potentially save more lives and improve the conditions of life for even more people, attract relatively scant attention.[33]

The ancient Greek poet Archilochus famously observed, "The fox knows many things, but the hedgehog knows one big thing."[34] For the past hundred years, health policy in the United States has been dominated by the foxes. They know many things about US health care, its organization, and how it is paid for. Yet despite their expertise, they ignore the one big thing about health: *health care* is only one part, and not even the most important part, of a *health system*. The citizens of France, Germany, and Sweden are healthier than Americans because of those nations' historical commitment to improve the social determinants of health. The social determinants are shaped by distributions of power, wealth, and income that affect not only one's access to quality health care but also to housing, education, nutrition, employment, transport, a healthful environment, and financial security. They include not only built environments, such as schools, workplaces, public spaces, and transportation networks, but also the power structures that create the opportunities to live a healthy life.[35] *Health care*, on the other hand, is composed of all the organizations that deliver care and medical services, including hospitals, physicians' practices, nursing homes, and clinics, as well as those that arrange the financing of care, including governments, states, local communities, and private insurance companies.[36] The *health system* thus includes *health care*, but it also comprises the political, social, cultural, and physical environments that influence the population's health.[37] This expansive definition of a health system clearly requires a delineation of boundaries. That is, if so many things affect our health, where does the health system stop and the rest of society begin?[38]

My answer relies on history. The relationship between a nation's health system and the broader society is fluid and varies over time. For example, the churches of late nineteenth-century Sweden that provided sustenance to frail elderly men who had been involuntarily cast off from the country's factories played a critical role in Sweden's health system of the era. Without the churches, many more unemployed men and their dependent families would have suffered illness and died prematurely, driving up the nation's mortality rate. Yet those same churches today play a relatively small role in Sweden's health system. They have been replaced by income-tax-funded universal old-age pensions whose first iteration appeared in 1913. Yet both institutions—churches and old-age pensions—provided financial security, which is a key social determinant of elderly health. Nineteenth-century Swedish churches rescued the lives of many, but income-tax-funded pensions were even more effective. A historical lens permits us to see that many institutions and practices are implicated in health system change and effectiveness.

I call this approach historical health system analysis. Because the challenges to health are constantly changing, we must conceive of a nation's health system as eternally dynamic. It should be judged not only by the effectiveness of its health care component but also on its ability to respond to the foremost sociohistorical and environmental developments of the modern era: industrialization, urbanization, globalization, pandemic disease, and climate change. A good health system produces strong health outcomes by protecting and promoting health in the face of these challenges. This broad, historically informed definition of a health system diverges from that used by many influential US health policy researchers.[39] Their narrower, health care–focused definition hinders the development of a wider appreciation of the social determinants of health. Relatively few studies examine health system development over century-long periods. Yet the institutions that shaped today's social determinants can only be understood by asking questions about the past.

I chose the social democracies of France, Germany, and Sweden for comparison to the United States because all three—in different ways and for differing reasons—invented some of the world's most successful health-promoting institutions, beginning in the late nineteenth century. They also possess per capita incomes comparable to the United States and market-driven economies, albeit tempered by social democratic principles. France began building a family-centered social state in the 1870s, enacting successive reforms to protect maternal, infant, and child health. Germany created the first social insurance system for illness, workplace accidents, disability, and old age in the 1880s. To these protections Germans wed pioneering occupational safeguards and healthful labor market practices beginning in the 1920s. Sweden implemented the world's first universal, income-tax-funded pension system in 1913, ensuring elderly people's financial security alongside comprehensive health and long-term care services. All three nations have achieved universal access to high quality health care, an important social determinant in its own right. Yet France, Germany, and Sweden differ markedly from one another in how they fund their social safety nets and other programs to ensure strong population health outcomes.

These differences draw our attention to the historical resource allocation choices of American, French, German, and Swedish leaders. Sociological and epidemiological research attests to the primordial role that social safety nets and other health promoting institutions play in the improvement of health outcomes.[40] Despite their varying political persuasions, the leaders of France, Germany, and Sweden used their power to create effective programs to protect health and to ensure its equitable distribution. As the medical sociologists Jason Beckfield and Nancy Krieger put it, "Power, after all, is the heart of the matter—and the science of health inequities can no more shy away from this question than can physicists ignore gravity or physicians ignore pain . . . epidemiology and political sociology need each other."[41]

In both the European and the American pasts, reformers who wished to improve their nation's social determinants of health had to overcome powerful interests within their polities. For example, in the 1880s, a conservative leader, German chancellor Otto von Bismarck, took on his fellow conservatives and industrialists. They believed that the government should play little or no role in the relief of workers who confronted dangerous workplaces in the new industries of the era. In true laissez-faire fashion, employers preferred that market forces be left alone, regardless of the asymmetrical power relations between the fledgling workers' unions and employers. The success of reformers like Bismarck and many others described in this book resulted from their ability to *decommodify* health without interrupting capitalist markets altogether. By decommodify I mean acting to remove or diminish the influence of market forces on access to a healthy life. For example, German leaders deployed government power to improve the social determinants of health by protecting workers from the risks of sickness, disability, and old age through social insurance. In so doing, they protected their citizens' health from market forces, which, if left completely unchecked, would have ravaged the very worker productivity on which the national economy depended. Indeed, historical analysis shows that reforms that promoted health were essential to economic growth. Politics, not economics, were the grounds on which reform battles were fought. Poor health is not inevitable but rather the product of politics, specifically whether political leaders succeed or fail to wield government power to protect the citizenry's health and thereby facilitate national prosperity. The political power of the state is central to the analysis that follows.

The Importance of Government Leadership

There is a widespread perception that the state has historically intervened less in the development of the US health system than in Europe. Yet history reveals a more complex picture. At several critical junctures, the US government actively exerted its power, picking winners and losers, either by enacting policy or choosing not to. These interventions significantly determined the evolution of the US health system by making future initiatives more likely and foreclosing other possibilities.

Let me list five brief examples. First, since its creation in 1887, the US National Institutes of Health (NIH) has played a critical role in the creation of new drugs. In fact, 75 percent of the most important innovations in pharmaceutical therapy, specifically the creation of new molecular entities, trace their research to the NIH, not private pharmaceutical firms or funding from venture capitalists whose time horizon for return on investment is too short for basic research.[42] Second, for decades after its passage, the 1935 Social Security Act prohibited participation of agricultural and domestic service workers, thereby condemning half of the African American labor force to diminished financial security in old age, a key social determinant of elderly health. Third, the 1946 Hospital Survey and Construction Act, commonly called the Hill-Burton Act, gave grants and low-interest loans to finance the construction of approximately five thousand hospitals and clinics across the country, nearly one-third of the nation's total by 1975. It provided a massive boost to private-practice medicine in exchange for an ill-defined and difficult-to-enforce provision that these facilities provide a "reasonable volume" of care to those in need. Fourth, the 1954 Internal Revenue Service ruling that shielded employer-provided health insurance from taxation is among the most important causes of the predominance of private health insurance in the United States. The ruling, which remains in place, disproportionately benefited union and professional workers whose compensation included health coverage, leaving those in unorganized and lower-paid sectors of the economy with less access to health care. Fifth, in 1965, the US government created Medicare, which today provides health coverage to most Americans over age sixty-four, solving a growing crisis in elderly health. But it did so by steering the elderly, who are higher-cost patients, into public coverage where preexisting conditions could not be cause for denial of coverage. The creation of

Medicare thus permitted private health insurers to preserve their business model that relied on insuring a healthier, less costly population by virtue of their ability to maintain employment. Once the link to employment was lost due to retirement or disability, state-subsidized public insurers, either Medicare or Medicaid (and sometimes both), assumed responsibility for the nation's highest-cost patients. Even the most recent major health reform, the 2010 Affordable Care Act, which restricts insurers' ability to discriminate based on preexisting conditions, remains committed to the link between employment and health coverage, thereby sustaining private health insurers.

Notwithstanding popular perceptions then, the federal government has repeatedly intervened (or not) to determine the nature of the US health system. "States are lumpy," says historian Peter Baldwin to capture the concept that governments "may not be consistently laissez-faire or interventionist but be so in one respect and the opposite in another." For example, the United States has set the global standard on protections for the disabled and the enforcement of building standards that assure their access. American municipalities were likewise a decade ahead of European cities in the protection of nonsmokers from secondhand smoke in public places.[43] The question then is why the United States has been so active on some health matters but less effective overall than many other wealthy nations at ensuring its citizens' health. Is there a logic by which we can identify when government action is beneficial to health and the national welfare?

Economist Mariana Mazzucato's concept of the "entrepreneurial state" is useful here. As she notes, "Rather than relying on the false dream that 'markets' will run the world optimally for us 'if we just leave them alone,' policymakers must better learn how to efficiently use the tools and means to shape and create markets—making things happen that otherwise would not. And making sure those things are things we need." As measured by US population health outcomes, whether led by Democrats or Republicans, the US government has provided generous subsidies to market actors or protected them from risk in relatively ineffective ways. Social democracies, although not without their missteps, have been more effective through their attention to the social determinants of health, universal safety nets, and ensuring financial security. Also, rather than trying to pick winners and losers by subsidizing some market actors and relieving others of risks, European social democracies have more often sought to create and shape markets so that the national prosperity and health outcomes—"things we need," in Mazzucato's words—are mutually reinforcing.[44] In contrast, the historical record reveals that since the late nineteenth century, US public- and private-sector leaders have most often viewed economic growth and measures to improve health as mutually exclusive.

Let me be clear. US health outcomes have greatly improved over the past century. It is just that they are failing to keep up with the gains of similar-income nations in Europe.[45] In 1900, average US life expectancy was only 47.3 years. Today it stands at 78.6. In 1900, 150 babies out of every 1,000 live births died before their first birthday; today, only 6 per 1,000 die. The age-adjusted death rate, which compensates for the age composition of the population, was 25.2 per 1,000 persons in 1900; now, it is only 7.3 per 1,000. In 1900, the leading causes of death were diarrheal diseases and respiratory infections. Today, although chronic respiratory diseases remain an important cause of death, they have long been outpaced by ailments that usually do not strike until middle or old age, namely heart disease, stroke, and cancer.[46] In short, more Americans survive their childhoods to live longer and healthier lives than their great-grandparents could have ever imagined. Taking heart in these achievements, public health pioneer Charles-Edward Winslow observed, "If we could transmute abstract figures into flesh and blood . . . as we walk along the street we could say 'that man would be dead of typhoid fever,' 'that woman would have succumbed to tuberculosis,' 'that rosy infant would be in its coffin,' then only should we have a faint conception of the meaning of the silent victories of public health."[47] No one can deny the fabulous *absolute* gains in health that have been achieved since the beginning of the last century. It is the *relative* decline in Americans' health that is troubling.

According to the US Institute of Medicine (now the National Academy of Medicine), on almost every measure of health outcomes the United States ranks at or near the bottom relative to nations of comparable income. Worse, the United States continues to fall further behind other wealthy nations on most measures of mortality and morbidity, in all age groups up to age seventy-five, in males and females alike, and in virtually all other subgroups of the population. The relative failure of US health is *not* simply a reflection of higher levels of ill health among low-income

Americans or those marginalized by race or ethnicity. Even high-income, privileged Americans are less healthy and live shorter lives than their counterparts in comparable-income nations.[48] According to the Institute for Health Metrics and Evaluation at the University of Washington, since 1990 the United States has shown a substantially lower rate of improvement in lifting the burden of disease.[49] With the exception of cancer ("neoplasms" in chart below), the United States is failing to deal with leading causes of death as effectively as similarly wealthy nations.

Germany, in particular, is increasingly pulling ahead of the United States in protecting its citizens from death and disability due to coronary heart disease (CHD), a troubling fact given the proportionally greater resources expended by the United States to alleviate CHD.[50] Failing to correct the relative decline in US health outcomes would be to sentence millions of Americans to premature death, chronic disability, and suffering, a tragedy

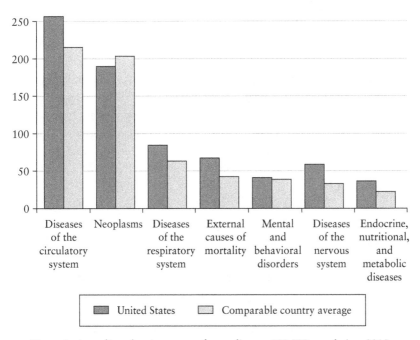

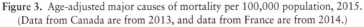

Figure 3. Age-adjusted major causes of mortality per 100,000 population, 2015. (Data from Canada are from 2013, and data from France are from 2014.)

Source: Peterson-KFF Health System Tracker, based on analysis of OECD Data, 2019, https://www.healthsystemtracker.org/chart-collection/mortality-rates-u-s-compare-countries/#item-start.

that is entirely avoidable with the solutions available in the twenty-first century.

The starkness of this reality underlines the US health system's structural violence. Sociologist Johan Galtung created the concept of structural violence, distinguishing it from personal violence. Structural violence, he says, is "the impairment of human life" by "ubiquitous social structures, normalized by stable institutions and regular experience." In other words, structural violence does not necessarily involve villains or even the intention to do harm. Unfortunately, the injury and killing, as Galtung points out, appear as natural "as the air around us."[51] What alerts us to structural violence in the US health system is the difference between *actual* and *potential*. The decline of US health outcomes compared to other wealthy nations indicates the difference between what Americans actually experience and what could be. By this standard, the US health system is structurally violent because Americans' regular experience of sickness, disability, and death are preventable in light of advances in similar nations.[52] Let us put this in terms of the number of years that Americans would have enjoyed living had the US health system performed like those of comparable nations. In 2015, 4,721 of every 100,000 Americans died prematurely before the age of seventy, a statistic known as potential years of life lost (PYLL). The average PYLL in comparable OECD countries is much lower: 2,723 per 100,000 residents. Which means that based on a 2015 population of 321 million, the US health system deprived Americans of 6,400,000 years of life.[53] Sadly, this preventable death toll has become dangerously normalized in the US in comparison to other places and other times.

The High Stakes of Health

I sometimes wonder if the relative decline in Americans' health points to the same kind of national fragility that contributed to the collapse of the USSR in 1990. At first blush, this would appear to be an outrageous question. The Soviet Union imploded from deep, structural economic and political causes: a rapid globalization of the world economy, fueled by advances in information technology, undermined the rigid, centrally planned Soviet economy in myriad ways. Soviet leader Mikhail

Gorbachev's reforms of the 1980s—*perestroika* (economic restructuring) and *glasnost* (openness toward new ideas and democracy)—were meant to invoke a transformation of society and politics from within that would permit the USSR to compete in a newly globalized world economy and maintain its superpower status alongside the United States.[54] Yet the Soviet Union collapsed quickly and completely in 1990: an event that the US Central Intelligence Agency failed to foresee. Indeed, the CIA assessed the USSR as invulnerable and expansionist only two years before.[55] But population health researchers, informed by their knowledge of the citizenry's rapidly declining health, had a rather different view of the Soviet Union's stability. Relying on data gleaned from international organizations and governments rather than spy satellites and intelligence agents, epidemiologists perceived a horrifying reversal in the nation's health that began in the 1970s. It included a rise in infant mortality and a decrease in life expectancy.[56]

What must be appreciated here is that the Soviet Union's health reversal came after decades of impressive gains. At the beginning of the twentieth century, Russian life expectancy and infant mortality rates were far worse than in western Europe or the United States. Yet, by the late 1950s, Soviet life expectancy, at 68.7 years, had caught up to that of the United States, and infant mortality rates had dropped below those of Italy, East Germany—the wealthiest of the Soviet Bloc nations—and Austria. The communists' massive investments in improving food production, water systems, and housing along with physician training and health care infrastructure had clearly paid off. But in the early 1970s Soviet health outcomes went into a tailspin. Death rates for nearly every age group rose dramatically above their 1960 levels. Infant mortality grew to three times the rate of western Europe's. The researchers identified heart disease, respiratory illnesses, suicide, and environmental degradation—all exacerbated by epidemics of alcoholism, depression, and alienation among middle-aged men and women—as the principal causes. Meanwhile, an increasingly dysfunctional and corrupt health care system proved incapable of rendering effective care or stemming the epidemics.[57]

Deteriorating health in the Soviet Union contributed to the rise of populist movements. So, when Gorbachev's *glasnost* reforms of the 1980s substantially lifted censorship, the people did not express, as Gorbachev had hoped, support for a measured restructuring of the economy.

Their message was rather, as political scientist Joseph Nye observes, "We want out."[58] Put differently, they wanted a revolution, which is what they got in 1990–91. If this were a story simply about how health researchers bested the CIA in foreseeing the collapse of the Soviet Union, I would not include it here. But recent studies make this tale chillingly relevant to Americans who are suffering a reality that appears fully comparable to what health researchers in the 1970s observed in the steelworkers of Kharkov, the collective farm-working women in the Ukraine, and the elderly men of the Soviet Republic of Georgia.[59]

Between 1999 and 2013, American white non-Hispanic men and women ages forty-five to fifty-four experienced a decline in their life expectancy. Their plight is reflected in the 2016 and 2017 national statistics that show a fall in overall US life expectancy.[60] This is highly unusual. It is downright hard in the twenty-first century to create a *decrease* in the life expectancy of a nation. Clean water, inexpensive food, modern housing, rapid communications and transport, and effective medical therapies make such a phenomenon extremely unlikely. The death rate of American white non-Hispanic men and women rose by a half percent per year, resulting in half a million avoidable deaths, a number comparable to the lives lost in the US AIDS epidemic from its inception in the 1980s through mid-2015. Like in the USSR of the 1970s and 1980s, depression, alienation, and drug abuse are playing a central role in the crisis. Chronic liver diseases and cirrhosis, drug and alcohol poisoning, and suicide were the principal causes of death. Indeed, some have labeled the victims as having died of despair. If that is the case, then a growing proportion of the total US population is similarly disposed. In contrast to European social democracies where suicide rates have been falling, the US age-adjusted suicide rate rose 33 percent between 1999 and 2017 to fourteen per hundred thousand. It is now the second leading cause of death for Americans between the ages of ten and thirty-four; and most rural US counties suffer suicide rates that are 1.8 times greater than those of urban areas.[61]

The falling life expectancy of non-Hispanic whites joins the chronically high mortality rates of African Americans and Native Americans who have long suffered from systemic racism. Life expectancy of black Americans is 3.5 years below that of whites; fully a third of the life expectancy difference is attributable to cardiovascular disease. Between 1999 and 2010, the African American population experienced over two million years of life lost.[62] American Indian and Native Alaskan life expectancy trails 5.5 years behind the US all-races life expectancy. American Indians and Native Alaskans exhibit higher rates of chronic liver disease and cirrhosis, diabetes mellitus, unintentional injuries, assault, homicide, intentional self-harm, suicide, and chronic lower respiratory diseases.[63]

Moreover, Americans of all races reported a decline in their midlife health status: increased pain, psychological distress, and difficulties with alcohol use and activities of daily living, such as dressing, bathing, and meal preparation. The effects of rising mortality rates and declining health will likely lead to a decrease in labor market participation and slower economic growth. They also indicate that a sicker population than the current elderly one will age into Medicare coverage. This will drive up the cost of Medicare to beneficiaries and taxpayers alike. Frustration born of poorer health may also help to explain the rise of anti-system, populist political leaders, just as it did in the USSR of the 1990s. The US health profile has stagnated to such a degree that it now resembles the former Soviet Bloc states of eastern Europe.[64]

Health inequities between population subgroups play an important role in national and regional health outcomes. Imagine two societies, one that is on average healthier than the other, and in both societies low-income households are twice as likely to report ill health than high-income households. Even though health inequality between low-income and high-income households in the two societies is *relatively* the same, the low-income households are better off in the society with the higher average health outcomes because *absolute* measures of their health outcomes are better. A 2016 study of health inequalities across European nations and US states found that population health and health equality go together. Southern states like Alabama, Kentucky, Mississippi, and Tennessee, where income inequality is highest, are also notable for their high prevalence of poor health. Indeed, relative income equality, high health outcomes, and health equality go together. Researchers concluded that if either a low-income or a high-income American could live anywhere in the United States or Europe, her health would most likely be improved or preserved in Austria, France, the Netherlands, or Sweden. None of the US states, not even those in which the prevalence of poor health and income inequality is lowest—Connecticut, New Hampshire, Virginia, and Wisconsin—would be better.[65] Even the best-performing regions of the

United States are relatively unhealthy compared to a large swath of western Europe.

Teasing Health from History

Although often difficult to fathom, health is an ever-present factor in politics and social relations. Bread riots and widespread hunger were common throughout France in the late 1780s. Even so, few would argue that poor nutrition single-handedly caused the French Revolution of 1789 that radically altered the course of world history. Yet most historians agree that the mounting health effects of the bad harvests and a piercing fear of hunger played an important causal role in the storming of the Bastille on July 14, 1789, a critical turning point in the revolution.[66] Also, lest we forget, the American and French Revolutions both began with disputes over taxes, without which leaders cannot directly act to improve the living conditions of their people. In the American case, the colonists insisted that there be "no taxation without representation." In the French case, the Old Regime's inability to justly reform its tax system created the crisis out of which the revolution was born. As the economist Thomas Piketty reminds us, "Taxation is not a technical matter. It is preeminently a political and philosophical issue, perhaps the most important of all political issues. Without taxes, society has no common destiny."[67] Americans and Europeans have long debated how best to pay for institutions vital to their health, such as pensions, health care, and education. Some choices have proven more effective than others. The argument here is that these choices should be judged by their outcomes, especially their health outcomes. If fiscal crises sparked the American and French Revolutions, subsequent events quickly took center stage—the Declaration of Independence, the Battle at Lexington, the trial of Louis XVI, and the rise of Napoleon. Health faded from the historical record, displaced by the high politics of revolutionary leaders and war. Health became contextual, less obvious, less exciting for historians to write about. But its influence remained ever important.[68]

The historian Marc Bloch identified the value of understanding common underlying causes between societies in his classic appeal on behalf of comparative history nearly a century ago. Bloch warned against a world where all histories are limited to one locale, region, or nation. He conceded that historians who specialize along regional or national lines are very good at understanding peoples and places on their own terms, free from any imperative to relate their past—or present—to some *other*. Yet with this practice of writing place-bound histories comes a danger. Authors quite naturally seek the causes and effects of the change they wish to describe within those boundaries. Much of the time they are justified in doing so. But in some cases, more general factors, ones that are shared by more than one society, go unnoticed. That is why Bloch advocated such a grand place for comparative history. Only through it, he believed, can we observe resemblances and differences across diverse lands and perceive larger dimensions of our common struggles that would otherwise remain unperceived or, worse, misperceived.[69]

The differences we now see between the health systems of the United States, France, Germany, and Sweden were not always so. Until the mid-nineteenth century, the leaders of all four nations shared many of the same reform goals, and the possibility of their achievement appeared similarly promising. Certainly the scientific and technological breakthroughs in medicine quickly crossed the Atlantic.[70] The causes for the relative decline of Americans' health are to be found elsewhere. Beginning in the late nineteenth century, US leaders responded differently than their European counterparts to the harmful conditions of life brought about by industrialization and urbanization. The institutions they created shaped the political, legal, social, and cultural frameworks that continue to dominate in the present. Historical causality can rarely be proven to the levels of certainty found in some of the other social sciences, especially those that rely on quantitative methodologies. There are many descriptive statistics in the pages that follow, but ultimately this is a work of history whose inputs and lessons require greater interpretation. Yet, despite its imperfections, historical research allows us to ask the biggest of questions, and the resulting knowledge is invaluable to our understanding of the world.[71]

Social institutions are highly "path-dependent." That is to say, at virtually every step of their development, specific conditions, values, and events exerted formative influences that in turn induced others. As each critical juncture passed, its outcome influenced subsequent change, making some results more likely than others. Political scientist Margaret Levi has aptly compared such a process to climbing an old tree. "The climber inevitably makes choices about which branch system to follow, and even though it is possible to turn around or to clamber from one to another—and essential if the chosen branch dies—the branch on which a climber begins is the one she tends to follow."[72] This metaphor applies to how a nation's health system evolves. It tells us that history matters, that singular historical moments possess tremendous explanatory power. But the singular quality of historical events does not mean that Americans and Europeans cannot learn from each other about how to solve their most nettlesome social problems. Indeed, the US Institute of Medicine deemed that "the United States can learn more by studying the policies that have been used by those countries that have been outpacing the United States on both health outcomes and social factors related to health."[73] This recommendation motivated my undertaking of this study.

Road Map to the Book

This book is organized according to the common stages of the life course: 1) birth and childhood; 2) adulthood and working years; and 3) post–labor market participation or retirement. For each of these stages I compare the United States with a different European nation: France for infants and children, Germany for working-age adults, and Sweden for senior citizens. Research from life-course epidemiology indicates the importance of the long-term health effects of physical and social exposures during gestation, childhood, adolescence, and early and late adulthood.[74] Working-age adults and elderly who live in France, Germany, and Sweden owe much of their strong health outcomes not just to the policies that have created positive social determinants of health aimed at their age group. They also benefit from the cumulative influence of institutions and programs that provided healthful determinants during their earlier years. A life-course approach embeds life trajectories in their historical, geographical, and cultural contexts, encompassing the myriad influences of the physical and social environments; these include the conditions of everyday life, access to health care, and the efficacy of public health.[75]

Chapter 1 examines French infant and child health programs that laid the foundation for France's family-centered social democracy. Throughout, I compare French developments with US policies and programs that sought similar child health goals in order to explain why the two nations' outcomes diverged. At its earliest and most fundamental level, health is the ability of a pregnant woman and then the mother and her newborn to withstand the stress of pregnancy and birth and then to thrive during the neonatal period, usually defined as the first four weeks of life. Mother and infant health are deeply intertwined; their success is substantially influenced by the familial, community, and national resources devoted to the pair's well-being.[76] The comparison begins in the 1870s, when France's infant mortality rate was similar to that of the United States. During these early years, French and American social reformers, physicians, and public health experts collaborated to craft policies aimed at the reduction of maternal and infant mortality, the improvement of child health, and the alleviation of disparities between population subgroups. Ultimately, though, France proved more successful in achieving and sustaining its gains in infant and child health, even as the country experienced dramatic demographic shifts after 1950 due to immigration from its former colonial empire in Southeast Asia, Africa, and the Middle East.[77] Throughout I explore what lessons American policy makers might learn, adopt, or adapt from the French experience.

Chapter 2 explores the institutions and policies that influence the health of working-age Germans and Americans. In the 1880s, Germany created the world's first social insurance for health, workplace accidents, disability, and retirement. This chapter covers contemporaneous US initiatives alongside German innovations and how social insurance affected the broader determinants of health. Work (or the absence of paid work) is one of the most important determinants of health in advanced industrial societies. The nature of one's work differentially determines one's risk of unemployment, which is strongly linked to heightened rates of mortality and morbidity.[78] Work also bears directly on health through potential exposure to toxic agents and other physical dangers. No less important are the psychosocial dimensions of the work environment. Substantial evidence links greater employee control of the workplace to better health outcomes. Conversely, a relative absence of worker power is detrimental to health. The development of employee participation in German firm management began in the 1920s, culminating in the Codetermination Law of 1976. That law mandates that workers' representatives fill half the supervisory board seats in all firms with more than two thousand employees. This chapter explores the links between German workers' enhanced psychosocial work environments and their superior health status in comparison to their American counterparts.

Chapter 3 investigates the health of the elderly in Sweden and the United States, focusing on populations that are no longer active in the labor force. For most workers in the United States and Europe the working years are followed by a period of voluntary withdrawal from the labor market. Sweden earned third place on the Global AgeWatch ranking of ninety-six countries. The rating considers health outcomes, income security, financial capability, and an enabling environment in determining the best places to grow old. The United States ranks ninth.[79] Life expectancy in Sweden stands at 82.4, compared with 78.6 in the United States. The chapter explores three social determinants that the World Health Organization has identified as the most important to healthy aging: 1) financial security, including the ability of the elderly to afford appropriate and safe housing, to maintain a nutritious diet, and to benefit from adequate means of transport; 2) social integration, the degree to which elderly people participate in the community, through continued employment, volunteering, or activity in sports, clubs, or other social organizations; and 3) access to preventive and curative health services, including long-term care, and the proximity of these services to the community in which elderly people live.[80]

An Old Debate and a Duel

Often lost in today's political battles over how best to improve and safeguard health is just how old the debate really is. In 1848, a Prussian physician who would go on to found the field of cellular pathology, Rudolf Virchow, traveled to the Prussian-ruled province of Silesia to investigate a typhus epidemic that had taken a particularly catastrophic turn, killing hundreds. Limited by the fact that germ theory was then still some thirty years in the future, Virchow's report to the Prussian government identified what were then commonly accepted causes of typhus outbreaks: above average humidity had created a typhus-laden "miasma" that entered the victims' bodies to produce the disease. But Virchow also introduced a new factor to explain the epidemic's high death toll. He called it "sociological." To the horror of the Prussian monarchy, Virchow insisted that the horrid miasma would never have killed so many had the Silesians been free, educated, and prosperous.[81] In a clear jab at Prussia's exploitation of the Silesians, Virchow provocatively asked, "How can prosperity be developed in a land which always gives up the yield of its activities to other regions abroad?"[82] Virchow thereby identified harmful social determinants of health in order to explain the severity and prevalence of disease.

Otto von Bismarck, then a young royalist politician, perceived Virchow's impertinence as an affront to Prussian honor. But because Virchow was a leading Prussian scientist and a gentleman, he could not simply be imprisoned. Instead Bismarck challenged Virchow to a duel. Entitled to choose the weapons, Virchow chose two pork sausages. He would use a cooked one. Bismarck's uncooked sausage would be laced with *Trichinella* larvae, the cause of trichinosis, a potentially fatal disease that attacks the heart, kidney, and respiratory system. Bismarck declined the challenge as too dangerous, effectively conceding the duel.[83] In this way, more than a century and a half ago, Virchow stood up for the powerless, directly attributing their ill health to their ill treatment by one of the most powerful nations on the planet. In so doing, he was among the first to assert that the people's health reflects the success or the failure of their leaders.[84]

1

INFANT AND CHILD HEALTH IN THE UNITED STATES AND FRANCE

All grown-ups were once children . . . but only a few of them
remember it.

—ANTOINE DE SAINT-EXUPÉRY, *THE LITTLE PRINCE*

Paris, France. I am standing at the reception of the École Maternelle André
del Sarte, a bustling preschool located in the city's immigrant-rich eighteenth *arrondissement* (district), trying to enroll my three-year old daughter. There is no language barrier. I speak fluent French. Nor is money an
issue. High quality preschool is free and open to all comers in France.
But there is a matter of health. A bespectacled middle-aged secretary pa-
tiently informs me that my daughter "cannot be enrolled without a *carnet
de santé*, a record of her vaccinations and health history." "No problem,"
I say to myself, as I hand over her multilingual World Health Organization prophylaxis certificate with all her vaccinations dutifully recorded,
stamped, and signed by various clinics. The secretary takes only a quick
glance at the document before saying, "Unfortunately, sir, this is unaccept-
able." I have lived in France long enough to know that failure to produce
exactly the right document makes protest futile. "Where might I obtain
the required *carnet de santé*?" I ask. "Your family physician or any *Protection maternelle et infantile* [PMI] clinic," she answers.

Little did I know then that "*la PMI*" would soon become a familiar term in our household. We also had one-year boy who needed a spot at one of the city's *crèches* (infant care centers). He too would need a *carnet de santé*. The PMI clinic on Rue Carpeaux soon became our regular doctor's office where the children always saw, by appointment and without charge, the same pediatrician who also had a private practice elsewhere in the city. Not only did our children need their WHO records transferred to a *carnet de santé*; they needed tuberculosis vaccinations (not just TB tests) that are not commonly administered in the United States, well-child visits, and occasional curative care. The PMI provides free preventive and primary care services to women up to age fifty and any child under six years of age, no questions asked, and its precepts are fully integrated into the nation's maternity leave programs, infant and childcare services, and preschools. In France, women and children are guaranteed access to the PMI because they are women and children. Comparable efforts in the United States rely on a jumble of federally assisted state efforts, primarily Medicaid, the Women, Infants, and Children (WIC) program, Temporary Assistance for Needy Families (TANF), and the Supplemental Nutrition Assistance Program (SNAP). Eligibility for all of them is tied to poverty assistance; therefore a child's access to care can fluctuate from one month to the next according to family income. Moreover, US children's health efforts are poorly integrated, if at all, with maternity leave programs, the federal Family and Medical Leave Act, childcare centers, and preschools, all of which are vital social determinants of child wellness.

In contrast, the French maternal and child health programs, although not without their problems, at least function as a coordinated whole. How did such a comprehensive system to protect maternal and child health come about in France? And what explains the divergence, which began in the early 1900s, between the US and French efforts to protect infant and child health? This chapter traces the historical development of the institutions that affect children's health in France. These include the early regulation of infant care and milk processing; the building of infant care centers and public preschools; the establishment of universal access to maternal, well-woman, and pediatric care; and the implementation of paid parental leave. Alongside the French story, I examine comparable US initiatives, which more often than not were vanquished by powerful entrenched interests or ran aground on the shoals of political inertia. The US initiatives included state pensions to low-income mothers so they could remain at home with their young children; universal access to children's health services; and subsidies for women to obtain obstetrical and perinatal care.

The United Nations considers the infant mortality rate as the "measure of all things" because it is "directly affected by the income and education of parents, the prevalence of malnutrition and disease, the availability of clean water and safe sanitation, the efficacy of health services, and the health and status of women."[1] The infant mortality rate is defined as the annual number of infants per 1,000 live births who die during their first year of life. An Institute of Medicine study that compared the United States with sixteen peer-income nations, including France, found that American infants and children, from birth to age four, are most likely to die or suffer from life-threatening conditions. The United States ranked last in infant mortality (5.8 per 1,000), last in neonatal mortality (4.4 per 1,000), last in low birth weight (8.2 per 1,000) and thirteenth in perinatal mortality (6.6 per 1,000).[2] The US child relative income poverty rate (20.9 percent) is much higher than that of similar-income nations (13.1 percent) and nearly double that of French children (11.5 percent).[3] US adolescents are also more prone to experience obesity, HIV infection, injury, assault from firearms, and pregnancy. American pregnant and postnatal women are in similar straits. Unlike that of any other wealthy nation, US maternal mortality has been rising for the past fifteen years, and it now stands at 26.4 per 100,000 births; in France the rate has been falling and now stands at 7.8 per 100,000.[4] Had the United States achieved just the average childhood mortality rate of comparable-income nations, 600,000 lives could have been saved between 1961 and 2010.[5]

Like the United States, France is a socially, ethnically, and racially diverse nation with high rates of in-migration from its former colonies in North Africa and Asia. In 2015, 12.1 percent of the French population and 14.5 percent of the US population were made up of international migrant stock. Yet France's average infant mortality rate (3.8 per 1,000) is below the rate of one of the most advantaged US population subgroups: non-Hispanic white women (5.6 per 1,000).[6] Educational attainment, an important marker of socioeconomic status, also fails to explain the relatively poor US performance. Infants of college-educated American mothers with sixteen or more years of education are more likely to die before their first birthday (4.2 per 1,000) than an infant from an average French mother (3.8 per 1,000).[7]

For much of the last century and a half, France and the United States successfully reduced their infant mortality rates, despite the world wars of 1914–18 and 1939–45 and the Great Depression of the 1930s. Indeed, in no small measure, the absence of war on the US homeland contributed to Americans' ability to outdistance their French allies in the battle to improve infant survival and child wellness during the first half of the twentieth century. However, by the early 1960s the US advantage in infant mortality rates and child health outcomes had evaporated. Then, beginning in the 1970s, quite to the surprise of American health experts, other wealthy nations, including France, surpassed the United States. The Americans have since fallen further behind with each passing year.[8]

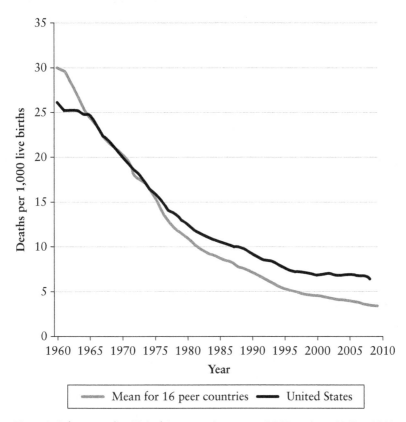

Figure 4. Infant mortality: United States vs. sixteen peer OECD nations, 1960 to 2009.

Source: National Research Council and Institute of Medicine, *U.S. Health in International Perspective: Shorter Lives, Poorer Health*, ed. Steven H. Woolf and Laudan Aron (Washington, DC: National Academies Press, 2013), 68.

This chapter identifies three historical developments that together explain why the French health system became more effective than the US health system at protecting infant and child health. First, the federal structure of the US government under which states could ignore or block national initiatives impeded child health efforts until the mid-twentieth century. Prior to the 1930s, the Supreme Court's interpretation of the Constitution restricted federal government actions on health and welfare matters, reserving those for the states. In contrast, the French Republic possesses a unified national government whose sovereignty over social policy matters is wide-ranging. Second, US private-practice physicians highhandedly mistook the power of their profession for an effective health system and blocked all government efforts to create universal access to health care services, including those specifically focused on children. French doctors also opposed state intervention into health care but ultimately struck a grand bargain with legislators that permitted the establishment of universal health care while protecting fee-for-service medicine and physicians' professional sovereignty. Third, the United States deployed means-tested social and health care services, which, when joined with the heavy reliance on employer-based health coverage, created a tragic (and absurd) dichotomy between "deserving" and "less deserving" children. France reserved some of its social services for low-income families, but most maternal, infant, and child health programs are universally available to all comers.

The State, Race, and Class

The federal structure of the US government prevented laws passed in Washington, DC, from being imposed on the states until the 1930s, hindering US progress on infant and child health. Cities often stepped into the breach, implementing bold initiatives on behalf of their youngest residents. In contrast, France has long possessed a unified national government. Its regional administrative units, the *départements* and *régions*, although important in some matters, possess neither the political authority nor funding resources of US states. The national government based in Paris could move quickly, imposing its will on even the most recalcitrant regional political leaders. Its most important early success took the form of 1874 Roussel Law.

In the 1870s, a French country doctor, Théophile Roussel, who had been elected to the National Assembly, exposed the living conditions of newborns under the care of wet nurses. France's industrial centers were woefully short of childcare options, especially for infants. Eventually, there arose a private unregulated wet-nursing and childcare industry that annually accepted some ninety thousand infants and children. Nearly 10 percent of French children ages zero to five lived with wet nurses, and in Paris, half of all newborns were so cared for. To be sure, many wet nurses provided their charges with adequate, even excellent attention. But Roussel exposed others who proffered fatally dangerous environments, especially for newborns. Shortages of breast milk meant the substitution of adulterated and unsanitary cow's milk; too often the homes lacked sufficient heat; and the ignorance or willful disregard of hygiene practices surrounding defecation and bathing made infection common. Roussel railed against the plight of the suffering children, whom he called "this human capital that is so easily destroyed."[9] France's Academy of Medicine had also been studying the wet-nursing industry and endorsed Roussel's bill, assuring its passage. The new law required public health inspections of all facilities that accepted children of less than two years of age for wet-nursing or care in return for compensation. It also obligated wet nurses to demonstrate that their own children under seven months old were receiving proper care.[10]

The 1874 Roussel Law contributed to a decline in infant mortality by 1915. Equally important, it institutionalized the nation's commitment to the improvement of infant and child health through the creation of a national health infrastructure. The government divided the country into public health districts; it developed standards of sanitation and methods for their measurement; and it hired hundreds of medical inspectors, drawn from local physicians who were engaged on a part-time, fee-for-service basis. The Roussel Law thereby created an expertise in public health administration that could facilitate subsequent health initiatives.[11]

Meanwhile, the United States took a different path that at first appeared promising. Health advocates, led by the New York surgeon Stephen Smith, founded the American Public Health Association (APHA) in 1872. Soon thereafter the APHA conducted a national survey of cities and towns greater than five thousand inhabitants in order to document local health conditions. In their responses, city officials commonly complained about courts' reluctance to enforce health laws, "lest they seem to abridge the rights of property and individual freedom."[12] Determined to empower local health efforts, APHA leaders appealed to Congress and to President Rutherford B. Hayes to create a national board of health. The APHA's lobbying effort succeeded in 1879, aided by the coincidence of a deadly yellow fever epidemic in the Mississippi Valley. However, Congress funded only seven physicians to cover the entire nation. Undeterred, the new National Board of Health forged ahead. Its first project was to create national quarantine standards to contain outbreaks of infectious disease. Immediately, several powerful state politicians objected. They refused to recognize any federal government authority on health matters and demanded the termination of the board. In 1883, Congress complied.[13] Not until 1912 did the United States again create a national health authority, the US Public Health Service (USPHS). Even then, the powers of the USPHS to coordinate state health laws, let alone enforce national measures, paled compared to France's Ministry of Health. When the US Public Health Service finally succeeded at overseeing infant and child health measures, it relegated immigrants and nonwhites to lower standards rather than ensuring broad-based efforts for all children.

Indeed, social Darwinism and eugenics colored US child health efforts from the beginning. The National Eugenics Society, led by Yale economist Irving Fisher, insisted that public health officials needed to first preserve what he called the "vitality of the national stock," by which he meant northern and western European white Americans.[14] Early US public health officials established the practice of analyzing infant mortality by race and ethnicity, ignoring socioeconomic class, and focusing most of their attention on recent immigrants. This opened the way to nativist, pseudoscientific, racist interpretations that ascribed infant mortality differentials between whites and nonwhites to biological determinism about which public health agents believed nothing could be done. Indeed, the president of the American Statistical Association, Frederick L. Hoffman, denounced those who attributed poor health and infant deaths to environmental or social conditions, saying, "It is not in *the conditions of life* but in *the race traits and tendencies* that we find the causes of excess mortality."[15] The ability to appreciate the effects of racial and ethnic discrimination is vitally important in a pluralistic society.[16] However, the absence of analysis according to socioeconomic class hindered a comprehensive understanding of the social determinants of infant mortality. If US health officials had studied poor people, regardless of race or ethnicity, the full mix of factors that cause infant death and children's ill health would have become apparent sooner.

France was hardly a utopia in this regard. Many French leaders embraced hereditarian eugenics, a form of biological determinism. It espoused that laziness and mental capability were inherited traits; therefore poor and working-class people were entirely responsible for their own ill health and poverty. Ultimately, though, public health officials who persisted in such beliefs could not remain in their positions when the power of workers' unions and the Socialist Party increased. Together they advocated improved sanitation, social insurance, and better access to health care alongside their demands for higher wages and better working conditions.[17] Such political clout would elude racial and ethnic minorities in the United States until the civil rights movement in the second half of the twentieth century. Even today, infant and child health programs in the United States remain burdened by their ties to means-tested poverty assistance.

Milk and the Medicalization of Motherhood, 1890–1920

The quest for better milk and better mothers dominated US and French leaders' efforts to decrease infant mortality for three decades beginning in the late nineteenth century. With one notable exception, physicians were at the forefront of this quest on both sides of the Atlantic. Despite advancements in curative medicine, French doctors remained more committed than their American counterparts to improvements in the broader physical and social environments. These included the pasteurization of milk, paid maternal leave, and access for pregnant and postnatal women to health services. This tendency, first visible in 1900, would ultimately mark an important divergence in the two nations' health systems by century's end.

Paris obstetrician Adolphe Pinard, who developed a technique still employed today to vaginally deliver breech babies, became one of the most important advocates of puericulture. Puericulture is the instruction of new mothers in science-based infant and child care. Indeed, puericulture served as the basis for the new medical specialty of pediatrics in France. The new pediatricians, virtually all men, deployed science as a justification to disregard women's traditional knowledge and the longstanding role of *sages femmes* (midwives). Pinard defined puericulture as "the science of hygienic and physiologically sound child care and rearing," leaving little doubt that men would dominate puericulture and pediatrics if only because at the time there were very few women scientists or physicians.[18] Although Pinard lent his eminent scientific reputation to puericulture, he was not its principal booster.

That task fell to Paul Strauss, legislator and sometime minister of health in the 1920s. Strauss's 1901 book *Dépopulation et puériculture* became the virtual bible of the puericulture movement. It stressed, "Infant mortality is overwhelming and disproportionately related to factors *before* and *after* the birth."[19] Strauss's explicitly perinatal approach, which focused on both mother and infant from six months before birth to six days after, diverged from contemporaneous US efforts. Americans instead emphasized postnatal infant health and were less concerned with the health of the pregnant woman and new mother.

Directly from the puericulture movement's concern for prenatal women came France's early commitment to paid maternity leave. According to Strauss, "If future mothers are overworked by excess industrial work, suffering a painful existence, a pitiful pregnancy, these unfortunate circumstances diminish the vitality of the feeble and dependent being who is in danger of being mortally wounded even before seeing the light of day." Strauss called for public health authorities to inspect workplaces and to set minimum maternity leaves that would be paid for by the workers themselves. He pointed to "women workers in dressmaking, embroidery, lacemaking, haberdashery, button and ribbons—[who] contribute on average three francs per year, twenty-five centimes per month in order to assure themselves a stipend of twelve francs per week for four weeks [in case of pregnancy]." Although he rejected state financing of maternity leave, Strauss stressed that perinatal medicine and puericulture were critical in the battle against infant mortality, writing, "Science has permitted us to prevent, that is, to avert deadly illnesses, a new duty has arisen, not only for individuals but for government. . . . [and] our knowledge of social hygiene must necessarily lead to the expansion of social welfare services."[20] This combination of state power and medical expertise enabled France to emerge as a center of innovation against the most common causes of infant mortality.

On both sides of the Atlantic, bacterial gastroenteritis, usually transmitted via contaminated milk, was by far the single most important cause of death in newborns.[21] Bacterial gastroenteritis manifests with vomiting, diarrhea, and severe abdominal discomfort. Cases in adults were usually self-limiting, but in newborns rapid dehydration and weight loss often resulted in death, especially during an era when recourse to intravenous hydration and feeding were scarcely available. Babies who were not entirely breastfed were particularly vulnerable during summer months when elevated temperatures and lack of refrigeration caused exponential increases in harmful bacteria in raw cow's milk during transportation and storage. The Paris obstetrician Pierre Budin noted, "Under the influence of the elevated temperature . . . [raw] cow's milk . . . becomes little more than toxic fluid."[22] Raw milk also carried risks of bovine tuberculosis, diphtheria, and typhoid and scarlet fevers, all of which were especially harmful and often deadly to infants.

In the 1890s, Budin advocated the creation of neighborhood *gouttes de lait* (milk dispensaries) where new mothers could obtain pasteurized milk, paying according to their means for single-meal portions, which dissuaded users from unsafe storage that could result in spoilage.[23] France's *goutte de lait* movement soon became a vaunted topic at international conferences devoted to the battle against infant mortality, including a 1910 meeting at Johns Hopkins University.[24] Although encouraged by the opening of milk dispensaries throughout France, Budin remained unsatisfied with the results. To be sure, the dispensaries appeared a likely factor alongside the Roussel Law in the downward creep of French infant mortality rates, especially during deadly hot summers, but they were not without their shortcomings. Budin therefore created what today is known as "well-baby care," which established the authority of pediatricians to supervise the growth and well-being of the newborn while simultaneously educating the mother (and sometimes the father) on home infant-feeding and care practices.

Budin began with his own obstetrics ward at a Paris hospital. His first rule: breastfeed if at all possible. This he enforced by keeping postnatal women with their babies in the ward for several days after delivery, during which time they were instructed on hygiene and other matters. "On a chart at the head of her bed she notes with interest the curve, which represents from day to day the progress of her infant's weight." Upon discharge, those mothers who were able to exclusively breastfeed their babies had to return only once every two weeks for well-baby checks. Others were required to return more often to obtain pasteurized milk in sterile bottles and to record the child's weight. Budin thus added an educational component to the milk dispensary, which he called "nursling consultations . . . really schools for mothers, for in them we not only tend the child, but we also instruct the mother."[25] Budin documented a 60 percent reduction in infant mortality among his charges and an even larger decrease for those infants who were only breastfed.[26]

That this further medicalization of motherhood should have occurred first in France is not surprising. After all, the work of nineteenth-century French chemist Louis Pasteur permitted the safeguarding of milk through rapid heating and cooling (pasteurization), which killed pathogenic bacteria while preserving other qualities, including color, taste, and milk's nutritional benefits, even though a full understanding of vitamins, minerals, and enzymes remained decades in the future. In 1912, France made compulsory the pasteurization of all milk intended for human consumption. Meanwhile, France's puericulture movement, launched by physician Adolphe Pinard and Health Minister Paul Strauss, privileged professional knowledge and displaced women's power over infant care. Given its greater expense, Budin's model of nursling consultations spread only slowly in France, but it served as a crucial predecessor to a massive investment in maternal and child health after 1945, namely the PMI clinics that cared for my children.

By the early twentieth century, two distinct models of fighting infant mortality had emerged.[27] The first, led by the French, relied on medicalized perinatal care and well-baby instruction that stressed hygiene and breastfeeding, wherein pasteurized cow's milk only replaced breast milk as a last resort. The second model, advocated by the Americans, also stressed medicalized infant care and emphasized breastfeeding in the first instance. But US doctors were quick to abandon their emphasis on mother's milk if the slightest social or personal circumstances warranted. In the words of the leading US pediatrician at the time, Harvard professor of pediatrics, Thomas Rotch, "Maternal feeding is far superior to any other . . . [but] mothers who have uncontrollable temperaments, who are unhappy, who are unwilling to nurse their infants, who are hurried in the details of their life, who are irregular in their periods of rest and their diet and exercise, are unfit to act as the source of food-supply for their infants. . . . [Their milk] will probably be so changeable in quality as to be a source of discomfort and even danger rather than the best nutrient to their offspring."[28] Given the irregular sleep patterns of virtually all newborns and thereby their nursing mothers, it seems that Rotch advised very few American mothers to breastfeed their babies. In contrast to their French counterparts, American pediatricians instead devoted tremendous resources to augment or to replace breast milk.

American opponents of breastfeeding claimed to have discovered an ideal modification of cow's milk to assure infant health, and Rotch played a leading role in this campaign. As the first president of the New England Pediatric Society and founding member of the American Pediatric Society, Rotch almost singlehandedly assured that a technique called "percentage feeding" remained a top concern of the American pediatrics profession during its early decades. Percentage feeding held to the premise that, "in civilized communities the necessity of supplying the infant with food not from the human breast . . . will increase rather than decrease our civilizational advances."[29] As a substitute, Rotch advocated that cow's milk be modified in the laboratory to replicate the constituent elements of breast milk. His and others' research revealed that human milk was composed of approximately 87 percent water, 4 percent fat, 7 percent sugar, 0.1 percent ash, and 1 percent casein. Cow's milk was similarly composed except for one vital difference: it contained 3 percent casein. This led Rotch to believe that casein prevented digestion of cow's milk, causing ill-health and a higher risk of infant death. He later added concerns about sugar and fat levels.[30]

If Rotch's percentage-feeding theory had halted there, it might have been possible (although still cumbersome) to produce what he deemed safe infant formula on a large scale for widespread consumption among working-class and disadvantaged women. But Rotch also insisted that human milk varied from mother to mother, as did the digestive capabilities of different infants. Therefore, proper percentage feeding could only be undertaken with full knowledge of the constituent makeup of the individual mother's milk and the physiological needs of the baby's digestive system. To prove its efficacy, Rotch joined with a Bostonian philanthropist who funded several new laboratories in New England, which, at great expense, produced infant formulas that were tediously calculated for individual mothers and their infants according to Rotch's methodology. Digestive disorders and infant mortality fell, and nutritional health rose among the recipient babies. Yet the low presence of bacteria in the new, sanitary labs was probably more responsible for the improved health outcomes than Rotch's percentage feeding method. Indeed, the value of percentage feeding has been roundly disproved by subsequent research. It now stands as a singular example of the medicalization of health whose expense and procedural requirements excluded the poor mothers who most needed assistance with preserving the lives of their infants.[31] Nevertheless, American physicians who led the new pediatrics specialty embraced it.

Medical schools across the nation added percentage feeding to their curricula. After all, it was good for doctors' pocketbooks. Percentage feeding necessitated that a new mother consult a pediatrician in order to ensure her infant's health; and it helped to make pediatrics an indispensable addition to medical specialties. Little heed was paid to the fact that poor mothers could barely afford regular visits to any medical provider, let alone the additional lab expenses necessitated by percentage feeding. Pediatricians who advocated percentage feeding were more concerned with the building of a middle- and upper-class clientele than grappling with the national scourge of infant mortality. Unfortunately, their pecuniary interests also drove research. Professional interest in percentage feeding distracted US medical research from the genuine challenges of infant and maternal health. There was, however, one New York pediatrician who saw through it all. To the exasperation of this colleagues, he hewed to the French model of infant care, indifferent to the criticism he attracted.

Abraham Jacobi had long been searching for a way to bring safe milk to infants of New York City's poor families. Compared to Thomas Rotch, Jacobi epitomized the out-of-step loner of the early American pediatrics profession. Indeed, Jacobi, a German-educated Jewish immigrant, could not have been more different in class outlook and experience than Rotch, the native New Englander and Harvard man. Jacobi had fled Germany after spending two years in prison for his revolutionary activities. He sailed first to England, where he lived briefly with Karl Marx, before continuing to New York City. There he practiced medicine and taught at the City University of New York and at Columbia; he was also a cofounder of the New York Communist Club.[32] In 1893, Jacobi met the well-to-do merchant Nathan Straus, who promised to help Jacobi improve infant health in the city. Together the capitalist merchant Straus and the communist pediatrician Jacobi began opening French-style milk dispensaries (*gouttes de lait*) on Manhattan's Lower East Side.

In 1895, Straus went further. He funded the building of a pasteurization plant, which further enraged Jacobi's colleagues who were still unconvinced of pasteurization's merits. They believed that raw milk could be certified to ensure its safe consumption by infants. They also refused to accept that pasteurization might not violate milk's nutritional beneficence.[33] Straus and Jacobi ignored the controversy and pushed ahead with their milk dispensaries. By 1903, Straus was funding milk stations that annually distributed four million bottles of safe milk to the city's needy families. What is more, his pasteurization plant and dispensary stations were emulated by philanthropic organizations across the country. A 1910 survey showed that philanthropists had created 298 milk stations in thirty-eight of the largest cities in the United States.[34] Yet, as bold as Jacobi and Straus were, they could not overcome the institutional inertia that slowed American efforts to ensure the mass availability of pasteurized milk. As we have seen, the division of the United States into semi-sovereign states that could reject federal government initiatives made widespread pasteurization exceedingly difficult to achieve, even had there been the will. This left safe-milk distribution efforts to philanthropic organizations and cities whose resources proved insufficient to meet demand. Jacobi and Straus's effort in New York City constituted the most successful effort anywhere in the nation. Still, in 1902, only 5 percent of the city's milk supply underwent any kind of heat sterilization process, including pasteurization, prior to consumer purchase.[35]

A 1907 international conference on infant feeding held in Brussels condemned the feeding of raw milk to infants and advocated pasteurization. That same year, Chicago and New York began requiring the pasteurization of all milk that had not been produced by cows certified as free of infection. The results were striking. New York's infant mortality rate fell from 125 to 94 per 1,000 within three years. Raw milk–fueled gastroenteritis epidemics that had occasionally rocked Chicago, especially during summers, ceased altogether.[36] By 1919, seventeen of the largest US cities required pasteurization of their milk supplies, covering 17 percent of the total US population of 106,000,000. Finally, in 1927, the US Public Health Service formulated the Standard Milk Ordinance that defined "clean milk," today referred to as Grade A milk, and the requirements of pasteurization. Yet because the Public Health Service lacked the power to enforce its standards across the nation, the pasteurization of milk did not become a normal practice in the United States until the late 1940s, some thirty years after France's 1912 law.

A comparative historical analysis of the milk debate and the medicalization of motherhood in France and the US during the early decades of the twentieth century reveals two undercurrents that would shape each nation's ability to protect and improve children's health in subsequent years. First, France's unified national government enabled the country to move more quickly on reform initiatives, such as the regulation of infant care and the pasteurization of milk. Meanwhile, in the United States, a relatively weak federal government could not prevail over state leaders' objections; cities had to act on behalf of their youngest residents. Second, less apparent but ultimately just as important, France and the United States exhibited different propensities toward prevention, private medical practice, and the relationship of both to state-sponsored social services. The economic and social strife that befell both nations between the two world wars (1918–39), accentuated the divergence in the French and US paths.

Care for Infants and Children, 1890–Present

Milk and the medicalization of motherhood were not the only areas of divergence between France and the United States. Other reformers understood that child health was vitally linked to housing, nutrition, clothing, and other dimensions of a family's overall standard of living. They sought with varying success to pay mothers to stay at home with their young children in hopes of improving the physical and social influences on health. But most of these reformers also had a cultural agenda. They wanted to normalize women's "natural" vocation as mothers to combat the first-wave feminist movement that advocated female suffrage, equality of civil rights between the sexes, and the freeing of women from traditional social norms. In France, the conservative reformers who wanted to encourage motherhood benefited from the nation's unusual demographic circumstances.

France experienced an early decline in women's fertility rates compared to other industrialized nations. Its natural increase in population, that is, births minus deaths, fell exceptionally low during what demographers call the transition period.[37] Indeed, after 1850 French fertility and mortality rates declined at approximately the same pace; had there been no in-migration, France's population would have declined in several years after 1900. These circumstances gave rise to a widespread fear of depopulation and a robust *pronatalist* movement. Pronatalists advocate population growth through policies that encourage the formation of large families and the lowering of infant mortality. The popularity of France's pronatalist cause also owed much to France's relationship with Germany.

Although France emerged victorious in the First World War (1914–18), the death of so many of its young men was profound and long-lasting. If the US losses in the war were considerable at 117,000 dead and 204,000 wounded, France's losses at 1,500,000 dead and 3,000,000 wounded occupied a different universe of tragedy, especially since its population was only one-third that of the United States. The public and leaders alike continued to fear Germany's larger population in the event of another war. Few doubted that if war came again (as many expected) it would resemble the First World War, and a similar number of young men would be needed to protect (and die for) the Republic. French children were thus viewed as indispensable to national survival; as such, they occupied a space between public and private goods. Anxiety about an insufficiently large population to repel a second German invasion colored France's national mood and influenced social policy on infant and child health in the 1920s and 1930s.[38]

A transformation in Catholic Church doctrine also inspired France's support for children and their mothers. Pope Leo XIII's 1891 encyclical, *Rerum Novarum*, explicitly called employers to pay a "just wage." Wages, Leo admonished, should not be decided purely according to the laws of supply and demand, nor did the presence of a wage contract necessarily fulfill an employer's obligation to social justice. The pope defined a just wage according to a gendered model of woman and child dependency; earnings should amply sustain a sole worker and those who relied on him.[39] *Rerum Novarum* buoyed the pronatalist and social Catholic movements in France. Indeed, a group of Grenoble industrialists, inspired by

Pope Leo's teaching, began paying family allowances (*allocations famili-ales*) to their male workers with dependent children even before the First World War. Family allowances spread quickly in French industry during 1920s but not necessarily for reasons the pope had intended.

The 1920s were a time of soaring union membership, a shortage of skilled workers, and galloping inflation. Social Catholic or not, industrial-ists throughout France adopted family allowances, not out of adherence to Catholic teaching but as a wage strategy. They found that it was cheaper to pay more to their workers with children through family allowances than to repeatedly grant wage increases to all employees. Employers liked this unannounced strategy because they could revoke the payment of fam-ily allowances, which were distinct from contract-governed wages, for any reason, including beneficiaries' union activity. This threat tended to di-vide older, more experienced workers (who more often had children) from younger, usually more militant, strike-disposed, single workers.[40] What is more, the widely held perception of depopulation permitted employ-ers to dress their wage strategy in the clothing of patriotic pronatalism. Union leaders bitterly opposed employer-paid family allowances, insisting instead on the creation of state-sponsored social insurance that included family support, worker disability, health, and retirement programs. But French employers opposed social insurance and instead expanded their family allowance programs to include a "stay-at-home-mother allow-ance" (*allocation de la mère au foyer*). It paid a modest sum to all work-ers' wives who renounced employment outside the home to care for one or more children under three years of age.[41]

In 1929, a prominent Catholic women's organization, the Union Fémi-nine Civique et Sociale (UFCS), rallied to support employers who paid the stay-at-home-mother allowance. Its leaders, Andrée Butillard and Eve Baudouin, launched a national campaign for its universalization to all employers.[42] A study revealed that 8,400,000 married women were pro-fessionally employed, which prompted UFCS leaders to argue that high female employment rates threatened family life as laid down in the papal encyclicals *Casti Connubii* (1930) and *Quadragesimo Anno* (1931). Ac-cording to UFCS leaders, "[The professional woman] too often gives in to the temptation of life outside, walking the streets where luxurious shops offer their seductions . . . the woman who earns often loses her sense of economy." French women, they said, were abandoning motherhood, causing a dramatic drop in family formation and poorer children's health.[43] Though moral arguments alone could not prevail, the UFCS campaign helped set the stage for government action when economic conditions shifted in the 1930s.

Legislative support in France for the stay-at-home-mother allowance increased as unemployment rose during the Great Depression of the 1930s.[44] According to one deputy, legislation was needed "to facilitate the return of the mother to the home where she has an eminent social responsibility . . . and to liberate little by little a certain number of jobs."[45] In 1938, the government made employer payment of a stay-at-home-mother allowance compulsory for all workers who benefited from family allowances. The new allowance was set too low to encourage in-home childcare by mothers or to significantly reduce unemployment.[46] Nevertheless, by universalizing the stay-at-home-mother allowance, France crossed an important threshold in its development of a family-centered health system. Beginning in 1945, family allowances and a modified version of the stay-at-home-mother allowance became core programs of its health system. A comparable movement, also led by women, emerged in the United States but with very different results.

Mothers' pensions in the United States differed from France's stay-at-home-mother's allowance in two important regards. First, the movement occurred somewhat earlier, during the Progressive Era of the 1910s, rather than the 1920s and 1930s. Second, the target beneficiaries were not married women with children whom French reformers wanted to stay at home to care for their children but rather single mothers whose children American reformers wished keep out of orphanages. Despite these differences, the comparison illuminates well the role of early women's political movements on behalf of children and how reforms, once enacted, fared in the evolving social terrain of children's health in the two countries.

The National Congress of Mothers, which became the National Congress of Parents and Teachers in 1924 and eventually known as the National PTA, was the main force behind mothers' pensions. Alice McLellan Birney had founded the National Congress in 1897 and gained the support of Phoebe Apperson Hearst of the Hearst business and newspaper empire that aided its rise to prominence. The greater pluralism of American religious practices made it impossible for the National Congress to strictly adhere to social Catholic doctrines, such as those observed by

France's UFCS. Yet, like the UFCS, the National Congress hewed closely to an ideology that defined women's principal identity as "loving, full-time mothers, devoted to raising their children to be Godfearing, solid citizens . . . through the principles they inculcate."[47] The National Congress leaders participated in President Theodore Roosevelt's 1909 Conference on the Care of Dependent Children. Roosevelt enjoined the attendees to find a way for each widowed mother to "keep her own home and keep the child in it."[48] US Progressives viewed the movement to pay stipends to mothers to stay at home with their children as a distraction from the main battle of the day, namely the passage of public health insurance. Its lead organization, the American Association for Labor Legislation, refused to aid the National Congress of Mothers in its state campaigns for enactment of mothers' pensions. However, in contrast to the major French workers' unions, the American Federation of Labor (AFL) supported mothers' pensions. Yet the AFL's support never extended to state-level campaigning and probably had as much to do with preventing women and children from competing with men for jobs as with ensuring children's health.[49] These handicaps make the success of the mothers' pension movement all the more amazing.

Prior to the 1930s, the reigning interpretation of the Constitution restricted the federal government's ability to act on health and welfare matters, and this included mothers' pensions. Thus, the National Congress of Mothers launched a state-by-state campaign, seeking allies wherever they could find them. Allied organizations included local chapters of the Women's Christian Temperance Union, church groups, and women's clubs of all kinds. Soon the mothers' pension movement overwhelmed state governments. By 1920, forty of the nation's forty-eight states had adopted them, a pace only exceeded by workers' accident insurance laws. And the worker's compensation campaign had benefited everywhere from the backing of unions, many employers, and Progressive social reformers.[50] However, in contrast to workers' compensation, which became a pillar of the US welfare state, home mothers' pensions barely survived the decade in which they were enacted.

The class, ethnic, and racial biases of state and local administrators played a major role in their fleeting existence. From the beginning, the middle- and upper-class women's groups who championed mothers' pensions had appealed to legislators on the grounds that impoverished single mothers were "worthy" recipients of state aid because of their vital role in safeguarding the health and rearing of future citizens. This purpose made its way into the mission statements of many state laws. Local officials could thus determine the worthiness of applicants based not just on their financial circumstances but also on moral criteria. The mostly white middle-class social workers who administered the pensions discriminated against immigrants and African American mothers. A 1931 study revealed that only 3 percent of recipients were black, hardly reflecting their proportion of the disadvantaged population most worthy of aid. Indeed, social workers routinely used a criterion they termed "Americanism" in their assessment for eligibility. It included whether English was spoken in the home, the nature of the house and its neighborhood, and whether the domicile was clean and orderly. Immigrant women who lived in substandard housing in outwardly ethnic communities often stood little chance of approval. Moreover, the stipends proved inadequate to achieve the goal of the program, which was to provide a salary comparable to full-time outside employment so that recipients could remain at home with young children. Many beneficiaries responded to the low stipends by taking informal part-time work, which defeated the program's purpose.[51] In the end, US mothers' pensions suffered the flaw that dooms the effectiveness of many means-tested programs: the perception of them as charity.

France's stay-at-home-mother allowance was universally available to all wage-earning workers with dependent wives who cared for children under the age of three. The stipends constituted a part of the family's earned compensation, not charity. In contrast, those who administered US mothers' pensions viewed them as poverty relief for "deserving Americans." This left the program more vulnerable to shifting political climates and the fluctuating financial health of state budgets. The National Congress of Mothers had proved its political prowess in obtaining passage of mothers' pensions in forty states. But its political efficacy did not extend to the building of a durable constituency to assure continuation of the pensions. Poor single mothers who were daily consumed with the struggle for subsistence lacked the wherewithal to build a coalition that might have permitted mothers' pensions to persist like the stay-at-home-mother allowance in France. While the US mothers' pension program is now long forgotten, France's family and stay-at-home-mother allowances survived. The French government took them over from employers after the Second

World War in 1945. In subsequent decades the allowances became available beyond the working-class families to whom they were first extended. Ultimately, far from constraining women's professional lives, which had been their social Catholic creators' intent, the stay-at-home mother allowance presaged France's universal paid parental leave, which guarantees women a right to return to their jobs after a maternity absence.

Like the stay-at-home-mother allowance, pronatalism also played a significant role in the creation of infant care centers (*crèches*) that dot France today. The 1897 Law to Ensure the Proper Organization and Function of Infant Care Centers resembled the 1874 Roussel Law that regulated wet-nursing. It assured a minimum level of sanitation and professional competence in infant care centers. For example, all cribs were required to be at least three meters below the ceiling, and each infant was to have access to at least nine square meters of free space. All centers were required to be well-lit, heated, and cleaned daily (including all cribs); the infant care center management had to include a physician; and at any time the caregiver ratio could not fall below one per every six infants under eighteen months and one for every twelve children between eighteen months and three years of age. The law also enforced particularly strict measures on communicable disease, vaccinations, and the feeding of infants, whether by bottle, with pasteurized milk, or their mother's breast. By themselves, these regulations to ensure child safety and health could not expand the availability of infant care. However, that expansion came quickly upon the outbreak of the First World War.[52]

The war sent many able-bodied men aged eighteen to forty-eight into the French army. The unprecedented conscription led to an equally extraordinary hiring of women to run the nation's factories and commercial enterprises. Indeed, historians often refer to the First World War as the world's first "total war" due to its complete mobilization of both civilian and military resources. Soldiers on the battlefront depended like never before on the women of the home front who produced weapons, ammunition, vehicles, canned food, clothing, barbed wire, and other essentials of industrialized warfare. Many large manufacturers created infant care centers on-site to accommodate mothers, but most of the new demand for infant care was met by the creation of municipal and church-sponsored facilities. The expansion continued in the 1920s and further accelerated after the Second World War in 1945.

Infant care centers (*crèches*) today meet 18 percent of the demand for the care of infants through age two. Trained and licensed infant care and childcare providers (*assistantes maternelles*), who provide care in their own homes or that of parents, provide 37 percent of childcare services. French parents or other family members—often grandparents—ensure the balance for care. This task is eased by the nation's universal preschools that are attended by virtually all children from age three until they enter elementary school at six.[53]

From their creation in 1881, the government charged French public preschools with spreading democratic ideals and teaching the French language to girls and boys. Democracy had only returned to France in 1875 after decades of imperial rule under Louis Bonaparte. At the time, most of the French who lived outside Paris and its environs did not speak standard French but rather a local patois. Most identified more closely with their region than with the nation. France's national government set out to build a secular, democratic, and unified nation. Public schools, including preschools, played an essential part in this project. The Catholic Church had traditionally controlled many of the nation's schools through which it exerted significant influence over society and politics; the nation's new public schools replaced Catholic school traditions with secular, democratic values.[54] Inspector general of preschools Pauline Kergomard distinguished the preschool from simple childcare. She also rejected the idea that a preschool should jump-start children's scholarly development in preparation for elementary school. Instead, Kergomard fashioned a distinct preschool identity and learning objectives. To this day, French preschools follow a national curriculum that is created by teachers and educational specialists. It includes only light reading and writing primers. Rather, through play, oral language instruction, physical activities, and the encouragement of free expression, the preschool teaches children to see themselves as autonomous beings.[55]

In 1960, 63 percent of all French four-year-olds attended preschool. By 1980, 100 hundred percent did so—and attendance became compulsory in 2019. In contrast, in 1966 only 10 percent of US four-year-olds attended preschool, many of them in the federal Head Start program created by President Lyndon Johnson in 1965. Head Start is only a half-day program and requires family income below the federal poverty level. Nevertheless, most research on Head Start and other preschools showed significant gains in health, brain development, and ultimately success in elementary school among preschool children. Such findings spawned a marked growth in state preschool programs. In 2005, the proportion of American children attending preschool reached 69 percent, although the majority of programs remained either means-tested or tuition-based.[56]

Despite preschools' proven health and developmental benefits, US efforts to deliver universal preschool remain hampered by insufficient resources. Meanwhile, preschools in France have become firmly lodged in the national education system. As such, they are now integral to national identity and the contest over its definition. Schools comprise a place where social equality and France's particular form of secularism (*laïcité*) are strictly enforced. After I obtained the indispensable *carnet de santé* for admission of my daughter at our neighborhood preschool in Paris (as recounted at the opening of this chapter), the principal invited me to her office so I could ask questions about the school's function. It was a friendly chat until I asked, "Should Linden bring a lunch to school?" The principal suddenly became quite serious. "Under no circumstances," she informed me, "should your daughter bring a lunch to school. It will be provided by the school cafeteria with no charge to you. If you want her to eat something different than the other children, you can come pick her up and take her home for lunch." My French colleagues later explained to me that the prohibition on lunch-bringing aims to preserve the equality between students and the maintenance of the public school as a secular space. Rich kids cannot flaunt their expensive edibles in front of their less advantaged peers. And the school could not become a place where religious dietary practices distinguished some children from others. A controversial national public-school dress code for secondary schools disallows the wearing of "ostentatious religious symbols," forcing Muslim girls to doff their *hijabs* (headscarves) at the schoolyard gate. In the instance of school lunches, our family chose to allow Linden to eat at school. The meals were always healthful and, according to her, delicious.

Health Services and Social Insurance, 1920–1945

The US Sheppard-Towner Act of 1921 (formally known as the Promotion of the Welfare and Hygiene of Maternity and Infancy Act) avoided the pitfalls that beset the mothers' pension. Crafted by Senator Morris Sheppard, a Democrat from Texas, and Representative Horace Mann Towner, a Republican from Iowa, the legislation greatly expanded the US Children's Bureau, which had been conducting children's health studies since 1912. Sheppard-Towner empowered the Children's Bureau to move from research to action on several fronts that affected infant mortality and child welfare.[57] In collaboration with state health departments, the Children's Bureau sponsored thousands of events across the country in the 1920s. It hired physicians—many of whom were women—to conduct prenatal consultations, and it sponsored public health nurses to lead child health conferences. The bureau even outfitted trucks, called "Child Welfare Specials," that served as mobile mini-clinics for children and pregnant women in remote, medically underserved regions. As historian Richard Meckel notes, "Minnesota and Nebraska targeted their Native American populations for special attention. New Mexico, Arizona, and Texas employed Spanish-speaking nurses to give lecture-demonstrations and make home visits with the Hispanic community. And the South, although keeping its programs segregated, for the first time tried to extend public health services to blacks."[58]

In contrast to the mothers' pension for low-income single women, Sheppard-Towner provided services to all comers. Children's Bureau director Julia Lathrop compared the bureau's mission to the state's role in education: "The bill is designed to emphasize public responsibility for the protection of life just as already through our public schools we recognize public responsibility in the education of children."[59] All benefits were universally available: conferences, consultations, educational literature, and preventive medical services. Ample federal funding quickly attracted state matching monies so that by 1925 Sheppard-Towner had resulted in the creation of 561 permanent child health and prenatal centers, nearly twenty-two thousand educational conferences, almost three hundred thousand home visits by nurses, and the distribution of over two million pieces of educational literature.[60] Sheppard-Towner successfully raised overall community health through its employment of local physicians, nurses, and social workers and via partnerships with schools. That the Children's Bureau became so immediately capable of such tasks is not surprising. For nearly a decade, it had been conducting diverse studies on infant mortality and child health outcomes, including international comparisons. The research

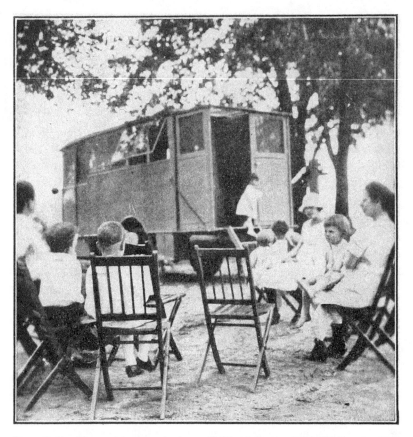

Figure 5. Families awaiting consultation at Children's Bureau "Child Welfare Special,"
circa 1920.

Source: US Children's Bureau, *The Child Welfare Special: A Suggested Method of Reaching Rural Communities*, Bureau Publication 69 (Washington, DC: US Department of Labor, 1920).

shows a sophisticated understanding of the social determinants of health, including the variables of class, race, ethnicity, and immigration status as well as sanitation and health conditions, housing, and the quality of milk supplies.[61]

Despite Sheppard-Towner's achievements and its strong support from state-level public health constituencies, the federal government soon extinguished the program. Although some of its activities would be renewed as means-tested measures under President Franklin Roosevelt in the 1930s, the Children's Bureau never recovered its previous scope or momentum.[62]

Two factors explain Sheppard-Towner's demise. First, its passage in 1921 had paradoxically occurred against a political backdrop of federal spending cuts and a Republican surge. Sheppard-Towner's success in the face of these trends was, in large part, due to legislators' fear of the newly approved Nineteenth Amendment that granted women nationwide the right to vote. Suffrage movement leaders had insisted for years that women, once enfranchised, would ignore traditional political alignments, focusing instead on issues that were important to families and children. Many legislators voted for the Sheppard-Towner legislation in order to prove their bona fides on family and children's policy to the newly enfranchised women voters. However, by the late 1920s it had become clear that women had not emerged as a distinct new electoral bloc; they had largely adopted the voting patterns of the male-dominated electorate.[63]

Second, the American Medical Association (AMA), already wary of Sheppard-Towner in 1921, organized against it.[64] Private, fee-for-service physicians viewed the success of Sheppard-Towner's prenatal and well-child clinics as a threat to their practices. Also, unless they were fresh out of medical school, few physicians at the time were trained in the latest and most effective prenatal and postnatal care approaches. Indeed, many practicing physicians learned about such care at Sheppard-Towner clinics and educational conferences. In 1922, the AMA's governing body condemned Sheppard-Towner as "an imported socialistic scheme" in order to tar Children's Bureau leaders as left-wing radicals who were somehow in league with communist revolutionaries in Russia.[65] It was an outlandish charge but potentially effective in light of anarchist bombings in US cities and increased labor militancy across the country. The AMA also launched an anti–Sheppard-Towner campaign. They directly lobbied the president and members of Congress, and physicians distributed political propaganda to their patients and state political leaders.

What the AMA disliked most about Sheppard-Towner was its guarantee of universal access to free preventive medical services for pregnant women and children.[66] Those services constituted a potential financial boon to physicians but only if Sheppard-Towner's provision of them could be stopped. In 1930, President Herbert Hoover sided with the AMA. On the subject of Sheppard-Towner, a White House statement announced, "Some activities now included in the program of most health departments can be transferred gradually to the general practitioner of medicine. In the interest of child health, insofar as practical, the family physician should become a practitioner of preventive as well as curative medicine."[67] But many beneficiaries of Shepard-Towner services were unable to afford private medical providers or to obtain sparsely available charity care. Instead, they went without the kinds of preventive maternal and infant care that were becoming common in France.

The AMA's lobbying campaign against Sheppard-Towner mirrored doctors' opposition to a public health insurance option for all Americans. US physician leaders not only claimed the right to define what constituted quality preventive and curative medical services, a claim that any professional medical society could legitimately have made. They went much further. AMA leaders insisted on the right to determine how Americans should finance and deliver health services.[68] Indeed, as will be explored in chapter 2, President Franklin Roosevelt's Social Security Act of 1935 originally included public health insurance that would have been paid by employee and employer contributions, much as Medicare is today. Yet Roosevelt was forced to strip health insurance from the bill when it became clear that the AMA's opposition threatened congressional approval of the entire bill. Therein lies a great contrast between the development of US and French health services for mothers and children.

This is not to say that French doctors quietly acquiesced in the creation of France's public health insurance program. Far from it. For ten years, beginning in 1920, a contentious debate over whether to institute public health insurance wracked French politics. Ultimately, the nation's largest medical association, the Confédération des Syndicats Médicaux Français (CSMF) proposed a grand bargain that tipped the balance in favor of reform. French doctors agreed to public health insurance but only if the legislation included a "medical charter," a sort of constitution that protected 1) a patient's choice of doctor; 2) a doctor's freedom to set fees; 3) the direct payment of those fees; 4) a physician's freedoms of diagnosis and therapy; and 5) the confidentiality of the doctor-patient relationship. France's 1930 social insurance legislation included the medical charter and quickly gained passage. It thereby established a framework based on common ideals under which health care would be extended to ever greater portions of the population.[69] To be sure, doctors, reformers, unions, government officials, and many others fought fiercely for advantage in subsequent years, but the law firmly established private-practice, fee-for-service medicine as the law of the land and confirmed its place in France's health system. Thereafter, France never considered a British-style National Health Service under which most medical providers are employed by the government. Nor has France ever contemplated returning to the era prior to public health insurance when so many went without care. A public insurer (Sécurité Sociale) universally provides substantial base coverage, paying 80 percent of the cost for most ambulatory care services. Additional coverage for the remaining 20 percent of expenses may be purchased from the country's many commercial and not-for-profit insurers (*mutuelles*). Some 90 percent of the French population possesses this complementary health coverage, either through their employers or through individual purchase.

Meanwhile, American physicians refused to negotiate a comparable grand bargain. Instead, the AMA adopted a purist's position. They zealously fought the slightest government intervention into medicine, fearful that any public program—be it Sheppard-Towner in 1920, the Social Security Act's health insurance provision in 1935, or Medicare in 1965—represented the proverbial camel's nose in the tent that would eventually result in a complete government takeover of health care. In contrast, France's 1930 medical charter appears to have inoculated the French against American-style fears of socialized medicine. Thus, in 1945, when the French government proposed a state-sponsored program aimed specifically at maternal and child health, physicians viewed it as an invitation to negotiations, tough at times to be sure, but not, as it would have been perceived by American doctors, as a declaration of war against their profession.

Child Health Services, 1940–Present

The creation in November 1945 of France's flagship program to improve maternal and child health, the *Protection maternelle infantile*, came two weeks after a reaffirmation of the 1930 medical charter that protected private-practice medicine.[70] The urgency of a program like the PMI was plain for all to see. The Second World War had caused deprivations of food, medicine, and other supplies essential to population health. Infant mortality rose 20 percent during 1941–44, childhood disease and malnutrition were widespread, and the country suffered a general decline in sanitation, housing, and financial security.[71] Indeed, General Charles de Gaulle, the unquestioned leader of a France recently liberated from Nazi Germany, called for "reducing our absurd levels of infant and child mortality." And, repeating the nation's longstanding fears of depopulation, de Gaulle announced, "France must have twelve million beautiful babies in the next ten years."[72] The PMI embodied the nation's effort toward those ends.

The creation of the PMI in 1945 marked an important milestone in France's transition from poverty assistance to universal protection, an evolution that has yet to occur in the United States. From the outset, the PMI offered its services to the entire population. The sole criteria for eligibility were impending or actual motherhood or simply being a child. The French Ministry of Health built PMI clinics and infant care and toddler centers (*crèches*) throughout the country according to population density.[73] PMI centers for prenatal care each served twenty thousand inhabitants; nursing and infant care education centers were built for every eight thousand residents. The centers emphasized nutritional diets for pregnant women and infants, the prevention of illnesses associated with gestation, the avoidance of maternal accidents and premature births, and vaccinations. The PMI dubbed this set of measures its "total health" approach. The perinatal period, usually defined as the period six months before to six days after birth, attracted particular attention. The "total health" approach also included a "whole mother-child-home" emphasis. PMI social workers, trained in puericulture, visited pregnant women and families in their homes to discuss infant feeding and safety. The PMI struck partnerships with private-sector actors that continue in the present. These include the contracting of private-practice physicians to round out clinical coverage at PMI centers. The PMI also hired full-time certified nurse midwives (CNM) on a large scale but also assured part-time positions for CNMs who wished to remain primarily in private practice. By partnering with local private-practice medical providers, the PMI effectively blurred the line between "public" and "private" even as financing became fully public.

What is more, the 1945 PMI legislation compelled medical visits for expecting mothers and their children, including ten prenatal exams and periodic well-woman and well-child exams after birth. All requirements of the law could be fulfilled at a PMI clinic or the family's private doctor (the latter paid for by public health insurance). Thus, again, private-practice doctors benefited from the state's entry into maternal and child health through increased traffic into their offices.[74] Beginning in 1970, well-child visits had to be recorded in the child's health record (*carnet de santé*), and that health record became indispensable for enrollment in all child-care centers, preschools, and schools. By 1980, the *carnet de santé* had grown to eighty pages; it included characteristics that in the United States would only be found in a well-kept medical chart. These included a family medical history, the nature of labor and delivery, the results of sixteen well-child visits from birth to age twenty, growth charts, a vaccination record, and summaries of any medical procedures or hospitalizations (or both). Private physicians who provide care to children must submit three certificates for their patients to the PMI. These summarize exam results at successive milestones of child growth: neonatal, month nine, and the child's second birthday. The data are anonymized for epidemiological analysis and population health research, a critical tool in the maintenance of strong national health outcomes.[75]

Cash support to families, pregnant women, and new mothers complemented PMI health services. As we saw earlier, the payment of family allowances, which began among nineteenth-century social Catholic employers and interwar industrialists, became universally available to all French families. The stay-at-home mother allowance was similarly revived after the Second World War in the form of the single-income allowance (*allocation de salaire unique*), which was paid to pregnant women who chose to give up employment during pregnancy. To these were added a maternity leave (*congé maternité*). It pays foregone wages covering six weeks before delivery and ten weeks afterward, based on previous earnings, and can be extended to twenty-six weeks in the case of a third child. The maternity leave program has since been extended to the mother's partner in the form of parental leave. Unlike PMI maternal and child health services, the new maternity and family support allowances are funded through contributory social insurance (*sécurité sociale*), whose eligibility remains linked to citizenship or legal immigrant status. France also greatly expanded its system of state-subsidized infant care centers (*crèches*) after 1945, which facilitated women's return to the labor force.[76]

In the 1950s, the government's multiple programs to support maternity, childbirth, and child welfare raised alarms of medical surveillance and control of women's sexuality. Indeed, during the immediate postwar decades, state officials used the PMI and associated programs to propagate long-held pronatalist dogmas, which included restrictions on abortion. Those efforts only faded after France legalized abortion on demand in 1975. Since then, access to abortion has been persistently liberalized. Public insurance began coverage in 1982, and a French pharmaceutical firm developed RU-486, an oral abortifacient that is 95 percent effective during the first fifty days of pregnancy.[77]

In fact, France's maternal and child health system today provides women substantial autonomy. PMI clinics provide family planning services, including contraceptives, alongside general women's health services up to age fifty. Laws also protect women's childbearing choices in the workplace. For example, employers cannot penalize a woman who takes maternity leave; pregnant women are entitled to job modifications, including a reduction in the work day, and time off for prenatal visits; and employers must provide new mothers with paid time in order to nurse their babies twice per day up to one year after birth.[78] Such protections facilitate France's strong female labor participation rate (80 percent). They may also contribute to France's fertility rate, which is the highest in western Europe (2.06 children per woman in 2018) and substantially higher than that of the United States (1.87 children per woman in 2018).[79] For a population to replace itself absent immigration, the fertility rate must reach at least 2.1 children per woman. Moreover, epidemiological studies indicate that France's maternal and child health system may be a causative factor in the extraordinary life expectancy of French women, eighty-six years, one of the longest in the world, compared to US women, who can expect to live almost five years less, 81.2 years.[80] As France was building the PMI, infant care centers, and associated support programs, the United States created two notable programs to protect maternal and child health.

President Franklin Roosevelt revived some of the Sheppard-Towner programs under Title V of the 1935 Social Security Act. However, in order to gain congressional approval, Title V had to pass muster with the AMA, which restricted its reach to economically disadvantaged women.[81] The Emergency Maternity and Infant Care program (EMIC) that served military families is a notable exception to the AMA's ability to prevent universal federal maternal and child health services. Assistant chief of the Children's Bureau Martha Eliot created EMIC to ensure maternal care to women who could no longer see their usual family physicians due to military mobilization during the Second World War. Under EMIC, servicemen's wives received prenatal, delivery, and postnatal care from a provider of their choice as well as well-child services until the baby reached one year of age. Only the four lowest military pay grades could access EMIC benefits, but wartime conscription and recruitment had so expanded the armed forces that the wives of 75 percent of the navy and 87 percent of the army were eligible. In 1944, the Children's Bureau announced that EMIC paid for one out of seven births nationally and operated in all but four states and Puerto Rico.[82] For many of these women, EMIC permitted their first access to hospital care and represented a major departure in the payment for hospital and accompanying medical services. AMA leaders conceded that EMIC placed them in "an intolerable dilemma." Opposition to improved health care access for military families would have appeared "unpatriotic." The AMA held its fire against EMIC until the end of the war and then successfully engineered its termination.[83]

After the war, the ascent of private-practice medicine and private health insurance, especially for curative care, continued apace in the United States. Preventive services, on the other hand, a critical component of maternal and child health, won relatively few resources. Big science, which had quickly ended the war in Asia with the atomic bomb, contributed to the orientation of US medical research. High-profile scientific and technological innovations in curative care became the highest priorities for funding, while prevention moved down the list. For example, the front-line public health workers who won the battle against polio in the 1950s attracted relatively little public recognition, while the scientists who discovered the vaccine gained fame and fortune. Between 1945 and 1955, when France was launching its PMI program, expanding its infant care centers, building preschools, and training and hiring primary care physicians, nurses, and social workers, the United States instead emphasized laboratory research aimed at curative care. Expenditures on US lab research increased from $28 million to $186 million per year in inflation-adjusted dollars.

In the decades following the Second World War, the AMA and the American Hospital Association also lobbied successfully for taxpayer funding to build new hospital facilities in which to practice the latest acute care techniques. The 1946 Hospital Survey and Construction Act, commonly called the Hill-Burton Act, gave grants and low-interest loans to finance the construction of some five thousand hospitals and clinics across the country, nearly one-third of the nation's total by 1975, providing a massive boost to private-practice medicine in exchange for an ill-defined and difficult-to-enforce provision that these facilities provide a "reasonable volume" of care to the uninsured. Hill-Burton included only token provisions for public health and the broader social determinants of health.[84] Those who argued for more forceful state action in health care and to improve the broader social determinants of health risked their careers by opening themselves up to being labeled communist sympathizers.[85]

By the 1960s, the only possible way forward on maternal and child health appeared to be means-tested programs. Sheppard-Towner stood as a martyr to reformers' battle with the AMA. The lessons were clear. Only limited expansions of state agencies for the provision of preventive and public health programs could survive. Proposals for maternal and child health had to be structured as poverty relief and their benefits tightly restricted to poor people. Any cash subsidies to families with children had to focus on the payment for curative medical services in the private sector. Failure to adhere to these lessons would invite a fatal attack from the AMA. The Medicaid Law of 1965 succeeded because it obeyed these lessons.[86]

Medicaid greatly improved access to health services for poor people, especially mothers and children.[87] Yet most state Medicaid programs also possessed the same shortcomings that hampered previous reforms. Compared to the French children's health system, Medicaid still overemphasizes curative care and is poorly integrated with other children's health programs, such as infant care and childcare centers, preschools, and parental leave. For example, the effectiveness of Medicaid's Early Periodic Screening Diagnostic and Treatment (EPSDT) remains hampered by patients' limited access to necessary exams and lab tests.[88] Medicaid also reinforces the fragmented delivery and varied availability of US maternal and child health programs due to its reliance on state matching funds. For example, one state, Arizona, did not even offer Medicaid benefits to its residents until 1982, some twenty years after approval of the federal legislation in 1965. Reliance on state partnerships also make the program vulnerable to funding cuts. As we saw in the case of mothers' pensions earlier in the century, poor families generally lack the time and wherewithal to advocate for public policy. The political weakness of Medicaid (in contrast to Medicare) has necessitated disparate legislation to provide essential services related to maternal and child health. These include the 1964 and 1977 Food Stamp Acts; the 1965 Economic Opportunity Act, which created community health centers; the 1972 Special Supplemental Nutrition Program for Women, Infants and Children (WIC); and the 1997 State Children's Health Insurance Program (SCHIP), which provides insurance to families just above poverty levels. All have suffered budget cutbacks during economic downturns due to tenuous federal and state commitments.[89]

Most nettlesome, the vulnerability of Medicaid belies the absence of a reckoning between individual liberty and social equality in the US health system. That is, Americans have yet to decide whether quality health coverage should be de-commodified and therefore available to all children, like public education, or whether health care is simply a private commodity, in which case the children's parents must earn it in the labor market. American families who enjoy quality health coverage for which they trade part of their cash wages see themselves (and are viewed by others) as responsible citizens who "deserve" the access to health care they receive in the event of an unexpected illness or accident. These "deserving" citizens are celebrated for their work and rewarded with health security. The ugly underside of this ethos is that many working families who lack access to employer-provided health insurance are viewed as "less deserving" of maternal and child health. Their only legitimate claim, says the ethos, is to health care for the poor, that is, Medicaid, or the hope of finding a sufficiently robust private policy on an Affordable Care Act (ACA) insurance exchange that has varying offerings by region.[90] If legislators had followed the more effective French model for maternal and child health, Medicaid would have been structured as a fully federal contributory social insurance program like Medicare, and additional child health programs, such as WIC and Head Start, would be fully integrated with it.[91] Evidence for the potential of Medicaid to improve health outcomes has emerged from recent studies that compare trends in states that chose to expand their Medicaid programs under the ACA.

Authors of the ACA sought a nationwide expansion of Medicaid in order to improve the health of low-income adults and children who had limited access to employer-provided coverage. They raised the income eligibility threshold to 138 percent of the federal poverty line ($17,236 for an individual in 2019). However, a 2012 Supreme Court ruling permitted state governments to opt out of the expansion (even though the federal government covered 100 percent of expansion costs in the early years and 90 percent thereafter). As of 2019, fourteen states, especially in the South, have remained outside the ACA's Medicaid expansion. These include states with large populations of mothers, infants, and children: Florida, Texas, Georgia, and North Carolina. The median-income level for Medicaid eligibility among the non-expansion states remains extremely low, just 43 percent of the figure demarking the federal poverty line ($8,935 for a family of three in 2018).[92]

A 2020 review of 404 studies examined the impact of Medicaid in ACA expansion versus non-expansion states. The subsequent published report offers compelling evidence for the positive effect of expanded Medicaid programs on maternal and child health.[93] The ACA requires Medicaid expansion states to cover essential health benefits, including pregnancy, maternity, and breastfeeding support, contraception, mental health services, substance-abuse screening, pediatric care, and chronic disease management. Many of these benefits are vitally linked to child health and the prevention of infant mortality. From 2014 to 2016 the average infant mortality rate rose in non-expansion Medicaid states from 6.4 to 6.5 per one thousand while it fell in the Medicaid expansion states from 5.9 to 5.6. Also, the Medicaid expansion states succeeded in reducing African American infant mortality at twice the rate as the non-expansion states. The 2010 Affordable Care Act Medicaid expansion is therefore linked not only to reductions in infant mortality but also to a reduction in racial disparities that have proven resistant to change for over a century.[94] Another study found that 710,000 children gained health coverage through what is known a "welcome-mat" effect, whereby the expansion of adult coverage led directly to coverage for dependent children. The authors estimate that an additional two hundred thousand children would have gained health coverage had all states expanded Medicaid under the ACA.[95] Finally, a 2019 National Academies of Science study identifies, "income poverty itself" as a major cause of negative child outcomes and notes that "expansions of health insurance for pregnant women, infants, and children have generated large improvements in child and adult health and in educational attainment, employment, and earnings."[96] The United States now stands at a crossroads in reform that could improve the health of mothers, infants, and children. In one direction lies large-scale change to how we provide health coverage through a rebuilt Medicare program that serves all demographic groups, what some call Medicare for All. In another direction lies a continuation of incremental reforms similar to the Medicare and Medicaid laws of 1965 and the 2010 Affordable Care Act. In a third direction lies political inertia, which would surely doom US children to incalculable suffering and unnecessary death.

Three main factors explain the divergence in the US and French health systems when it comes to protecting infants and children: 1) the institutional structure of the US government; 2) the power of private-practice medical providers in the US health system; and 3) the use of means-tested health programs, which, when joined with the reliance on employer-provided health coverage, created a brutal dichotomy between "deserving" and "less deserving" children.

The structure of the US government impeded national public health initiatives and efficacious social services. As we saw, state governments effectively blocked the creation of a unifying federal public health service until 1912, some thirty years after French legislators had empowered public health inspectors under the Roussel Law of 1874. Even though the US Supreme Court reinterpreted the Constitution in 1937 to permit an expansion of federal power over social welfare, federal-state collaborations endured as the dominant model for infant and child health programs. The subsequent federal-state programs that were tied to poverty assistance, such as Medicaid, failed to deliver improvements to children's health that matched contemporaneous French achievements. Poor women and children became but outcasts of the US health system, only able to access politically vulnerable and often inferior services.[97] It is little wonder that US infant and child health outcomes are poorer and falling further behind comparable income nations like France. In no small measure, the American Medical Association played a large role in this failure. Physician leaders repeatedly blocked state-level public health insurance initiatives in the 1910s; they eviscerated the Children's Bureau and Sheppard-Towner maternal and child health programs of the 1920s; and they thwarted well-developed plans to include health coverage in the 1935 Social Security Act. In contrast, French physicians ultimately reached a grand bargain with legislators on the creation a public-private mix of health coverage, which is far from perfect, but its performance as measured by population health outcomes, cost, and patient satisfaction far exceed the US system.[98]

Symbolic of the contrast between the French and US children's health systems is France's purchase of American neonatal intensive-care incubators in the 1960s.[99] The incubator had been invented in France in the mid-nineteenth century, and French obstetricians fashioned several variations of the device in the succeeding decades. Yet incubator technology never attracted substantial investment from France's private sector or government. Instead, the nation prioritized the broader social determinants of health: maternal, infant, and child care; preschools; maternity leave; well-child care; and preventive medicine. After all, incubators could be imported from the United States, while the improvement in the social determinants of health could not. In the United States, neonatal intensive-care incubators that served the well-insured, mostly white middle and upper classes substituted for the arduous task of improving the broad influences on health of all the nation's children. Harvard pediatrician Thomas Rotch stands as an early indication of this trend. His inane quest for the "right" infant formula embodied the US overreliance on technical solutions. Fifty years later the Hill-Burton Act similarly unleashed a massive expenditure on medical infrastructure that ignored a sensible balance between curative and preventive measures. By the 1970s, France's superior infant and child health outcomes demonstrated the value of a health system's attention to the broad social determinants of health.

2

WORKERS' HEALTH IN THE UNITED STATES AND GERMANY

> Legislative reform and revolution are not different methods of
> historic development that can be picked out at pleasure from the
> counter of history, just as one chooses hot or cold sausages.
> —ROSA LUXEMBURG, *REFORM OR REVOLUTION*

Kufstein, Austria. I am standing in front of my friend's electrical appliance shop in this Tyrolian town at the German border, site of a tête à tête between Adolf Hitler and Benito Mussolini in 1938. Brightly lit lamps of numerous styles beam onto the sidewalk through the shop window as the day turns to dusk. I enter and meander across the showroom to the store's rear where I enter a workshop. Technicians hover over appliances in various states of disassembly and repair. Karl, who served in the German army during the Second World War, founded this store in 1950. His eldest son, Dieter, now runs the thriving business. Equally as heartening as Dieter's accomplishment is the success of Karl's daughter, Ursula. She too inherited her father's penchant for all things electrical and mechanical. In 1992, she cofounded a small manufacturing firm just a mile away. If Deiter's success represents the sustainability of technical expertise at the local level, Ursula's represents the sustainability of manufacturing itself in Austria and Germany. Companies such as hers continue to play a major role in the prosperity and health of these nations. Given their unique characteristics,

even Anglophone economists call these small- and medium-size manufacturing firms by their German name—*Mittelstand*. They are innovative,
highly specialized, invest heavily in their workforces, and possess family-
like corporate cultures devoted to long-term profitability rather than the
chasing of quarterly earnings. In return, the *Mittelstand* benefit from their
nation's investment in the social determinants of health, such as efficient
social insurance, universal health care, quality education, and apprentice-
ships for their employees. Ludwig Erhard, West Germany's economics
minister after the Second World War and the architect of the nation's economic miracle of the 1950s, preferred to identify the *Mittelstand* by their
values. He called them representative of "an ethos and a fundamental dis-
position of how one acts and behaves in society."[1] As we will see, workplaces of all kinds have evolved to play a vital role in preserving the health
of working-age Germans.

As capitalist industrialized societies, the United States and Germany exhibit social norms and values that revolve around production, productivity, and work. Women have long faced additional demands beyond men,
responsible (according to the reigning social norms) for both production
and reproduction, the latter entailing substantial unpaid work in the form
of childbearing and child rearing. For both men and women between the
ages of eighteen and sixty-four, the ability to work, compensated or not,
is generally viewed as synonymous with health. Common is the statement
"He can't be that sick, he's still working." Conversely, an individual who
is completely unable to work during her so-called working years is often
deemed unhealthy.

Yet, in reality, an individual's ability to work and one's health are
highly interrelated. One's work is just as likely to influence one's health as
the other way around. Work is the single most important determinant of
health outcomes in advanced industrial societies. It is the principal source
of income for most of the population, and it mediates an individual's in-
teraction with other social determinants that depend on socioeconomic
status, including education, housing, and access to health care services.
The nature of one's work also denotes exposure to harmful substances
and psychosocial effects on health. Equally important, one's work influences the risk of unemployment, which is strongly linked to heightened
rates of morbidity and mortality.[2]

Germany holds a special place in the history of protections against workplace risks as well as contemporary initiatives to safeguard health through work. Germans were the first to create social insurance that covered workplace accidents, disability, illness, and old-age pensions in the 1880s, decades before such programs were seriously contemplated in the United States. Indeed, Germany's pioneering role has long presented a historical problem. Why, historians ask, was a monarchy the first nation to institute social programs that ultimately served as a foundation of twentieth-century social democracy? More democratic nations of the era, such as France or Great Britain, might have provided more fertile ground for popular measures to alleviate the brutality of the nineteenth-century industrialized workplace. As we will see, part of the answer to this paradox lies in the particular political machinations underway in Germany in the 1880s. However, another important part of the answer is Germany's long-standing commitment to safeguarding its economic competitiveness, which can only be accomplished with a healthy labor force.

Industrial working conditions throughout Europe and the United States were remarkably harsh in the nineteenth century. Workers' unions were weak, and even had they been stronger there existed little scientific knowledge or epidemiological data that could be harnessed in favor of workplace safety. German and American workers alike breathed particulate-dense air. Production processes used lead, phosphorous, mercury, and other toxic materials with little regard for their danger. German and American rural laborers and village artisans streamed into the growing cities to become the twentieth-century industrial working class, unknowing victims of the perils that awaited them. Yet German workers possessed a better chance of surviving the new industrial work environment because of the aforementioned social insurance programs that helped to shield them in case of accident, sickness, or disability.

Findings from life-course epidemiology demonstrate the long-term health effects of physical and social exposures during gestation and childhood. Which means that many pregnant German women and their children benefited from improved health insurance coverage beginning in the 1880s. Indeed, the effects of Germans' better access to medical care may have played a role in German soldiers' better health status at the outbreak of the First World War. Almost 50 percent of American draftees, all between the ages of twenty and thirty, failed their induction physical exams, forcing the US Army to create "limited service" categories for men who were insufficiently fit. As US army historian Sanders Marble notes, "Much of the problem was poverty and lack of access to health care: tenement dwellers and sharecroppers were often in poor health."[3] All German men were already required to serve two years in the military upon their twentieth birthday, followed by reserve service that included annual training exercises. Therefore, unlike the United States, Germany never conscripted hundreds of thousands of young men straight from the nation's farms and factories. However, we do know that only about 5 percent of twenty-year-old German men who reported for military service at the outbreak of the First World War failed their physical exams.[4]

Where do the health outcomes of German working-age adults stand today compared to their American peers? According to the Institute of Medicine, the health outcomes of Americans in their working years (eighteen to sixty-four) contrast sharply with their counterparts in sixteen similar income nations, including Germany, in four key areas. First, the United States has had the highest obesity rate for decades, especially among adults, beginning at age twenty, as well as the highest prevalence of diabetes and high plasma glucose levels. Second, the US death rate from ischemic heart disease (IHD) is the second-highest among its peer countries. Middle-aged American workers (age fifty) exhibit a less favorable cardiovascular risk profile than their peers, and those over fifty are more likely to develop cardiovascular disease and die from it. Germany, in particular, is increasingly pulling ahead of the United States in protecting its workers from premature death and disability due to IHD, a troubling fact given the proportionally greater resources expended by the United States on the problem. Third, lung disease is more prevalent and associated with higher mortality in the United States than in Germany. Fourth, older Americans report a higher prevalence of arthritis and activity limitations than their counterparts in Europe and Japan; both have been linked to a slower rate of improvement in the overall burden of disease in the United States since 1990.[5] These contemporary indicators of American health outcomes compared to Germany and other similar-income nations present two interpretive challenges.

First, our historical examination of the social influences on the health of American and German working-age adults spans over a hundred years.

During this period the causes of ill health and premature death underwent a fundamental transformation. In the late nineteenth and early twentieth centuries, workplace accidents, exposure to toxic agents, and infectious diseases, especially tuberculosis, were major causes of morbidity and premature death. Today it is chronic health conditions—heart disease, diabetes, and cancer—that comprise most illness and shorten the lives of working-age Americans and Germans. But these conditions only emerged as leading causes of death in the 1960s.[6] Unlike infant and maternal mortality rates, which have consistently served as prime indicators of children's and mothers' health right up to the present day, our health indicators of working-age adults must shift over the course of the period under study.

Second, the available historical sources lead our examination to focus on workers. Yet the health of the employed can only approximate that of the larger population of working-age adults. Moreover, who was employed and how intensively in the United States and Germany varies over the period of our examination. Women were systematically excluded from many jobs in both countries except during the world wars, when their labor enabled the continuation of industrial and agricultural production. Today similar proportions of American men (68 percent) and American women (48 percent) and German men (66 percent) and German women (46 percent) are active in the labor force. However, Germany shows a substantially higher overall employment rate of 78.4 percent versus 72.3 percent in the United States.[7] Historically and up to the present day, African American labor participation has been hobbled by discrimination and systemic racism. Also, the decline in manufacturing in some US regions has led to the early withdrawal from the labor market of many low-education whites.[8] As we will see, Germany began developing institutions in the 1880s that bestow substantial health benefits on adults whether active or inactive in the labor force. Comparable US institutions were either short-lived or made only intermittent progress.

Too often the relative US failure to create productive workplaces that also ensure the health of their workers is accepted as inevitable because of the American preference for economic productivity. Yet a comparative historical examination of the German case reveals the fallacy of this productivity-or-health tradeoff. German productivity levels have consistently matched US levels since 1950.[9] Moreover, in contrast to the United

States, the German manufacturing sector has maintained its competitiveness despite the globalization of industrial supply chains. Manufacturing still makes up nearly a quarter of Germany's gross domestic product (GDP) compared to the United States, where manufacturing has fallen to only 12 percent of the GDP.[10]

This chapter explores three interrelated developments that together help explain the divergence between the health outcomes of German and American working-age adults. First, early in its industrialization Germany adjusted its social policies and cultural norms to enhance the productive potential of its human resources. A limited labor supply in the late nineteenth and early twentieth centuries led Germany's conservative rulers to accede to the creation of contributory social insurance that helped to safeguard worker health. Meanwhile, mass emigration to the United States during the same period (from Germany and elsewhere) provided US employers with an ample labor supply. Employers could more easily disregard the health of their workers because it was relatively easy to replace them. Second, Germany's Social Democratic Party—the SPD (Sozialdemokratische Partei Deutschlands)—founded in 1890 and still one of Europe's largest socialist parties—became a powerful force for safer workplaces and more efficient systems of worker accident, disability, and health insurance. In the United States, neither the Republican nor Democratic parties were as effective in advocating safe workplaces or in the creation of efficient accident, disability, and health insurance systems. Although the Socialist Party of America's presidential candidate, Eugene Debs, won nearly a million votes in both 1912 and in 1920, American Socialists never achieved a national following on par with the German SPD. Third, Germany's social-market economy relies to a considerable degree on the successful collaboration between employers and workers. Employer-worker collaboration on health matters is found not only in collective bargaining at large companies but also at small firms where unions are absent. This is because German employees have recourse to "works councils" that enjoy broad jurisdiction over schedules, productivity measures, and the workplace environment in general, all of which are linked to improved health outcomes. The period of Nazi rule (1933–45) actually accentuated the state's commitment to worker health but only for members of the *Volksgemeinschaft*, a racially defined national community that excluded Jews, Sinti, Roma, socialists, communists, the "hereditarily ill," homosexuals, and others the state deemed "asocial." Instead of better health, the state imprisoned or murdered those outside the *Volksgemeinschaft*. Together, German developments over the course of the nineteenth and twentieth centuries, namely the institution of efficient social insurance, state actions to promote health, and local workers' substantive power over how they do their jobs, have resulted in workplaces that are both *physiologically* and *psychosocially* healthier than their US counterparts.

Creation of the German Workplace, 1880–1919

Critics of large state-sponsored social safety nets like Germany's often attribute their origins to "do-gooder" impulses that end up taxing people who work in order to pay for people who don't. Nothing could be further from the truth in the case of Germany. German social insurance was born of the same hard-edged political-economic philosophy that drove economic development on both sides of the Atlantic in the nineteenth century: productivism.[11] Productivism stipulates that a constant annual growth in productivity is the primary goal of socioeconomic activity. Depending on their circumstances, nations have pursued productivist goals in various ways, some more healthful, others less healthful to their workers. But in all cases, it fired the growth of industry and cities, and a popular fascination with technology. Productivism also recast individuals as consumers and, especially important here, hallowed the individual's role as a productive worker. As a result, work became normal and nonwork abnormal. Under the ethos of productivism, particular kinds of work were more respected than others. Compensated labor, clocked by the hour in the new factories, achieved a predominance unseen before in history, which led to a relative diminishing in the social value of domestic work and child rearing that was usually done by women.[12]

In dialectical fashion, German productivism's unrelenting demands on workers led directly to the creation of social institutions that were required to sustain economic growth. The nation's attachment to productivism is best illustrated by the career of Franz Koelsch, a physician and specialist in occupational medicine. He served under four vastly different governments from 1910 to 1955: the imperial state of Wilhelm II, the socialist-led Weimar Republic between the world wars, the Nazi regime, and the Federal Republic of Germany after the Second World War. In Koelsch's words, "The working man stands at the center of a purposeful economy. A people's wealth lies in the manpower and the willingness to work of the *Volksgenossen* [national community]. Therefore, it is our duty of far reaching and social importance to maintain human capacity to work and to keep it from harm."[13] Koelsch understood well the inherent dangers of the new manufacturing workplace where serious accidents and occupational disease were common; approximately one in ten workers fell victim to serious illness or accidents each year in some industries. Thus, a social norm, such as productivism, that demanded work from all able-bodied men could only be sustained if the state and the society made adequate provisions for the injured, ill, disabled, and senescent.[14]

Workers' accident insurance (known as workers' compensation insurance in the United States) emerged early in Germany as an indispensable component of capitalist industrialization and productivism. Similarly, health insurance became a necessity for the normalization of work and the achievement of productivist goals. Otherwise a bout of illness that deprived a worker of his subsistence could doom his ability to return to work once well. Last, the social expectation that workers were to fulfill their productive roles for the entirety of their able-bodied years made it imperative that the state provide a pension when work became impossible due to old age. The combination of these three worker benefits—provisions against accidents, illness, and old-age—constituted the foundations of the German welfare state. If workers were to be bound to their oath of productivity, in return the state and the society had to create institutions that permitted workers to recuperate from injury and sickness and to sustain themselves after retirement.

The nature of large-scale manufacturing and urbanization in the late nineteenth-century created working and living environments that sickened and hurt people. Poor ventilation in early textile factories meant that a haze of particulates hung in the air. Chemical plants and steelworks sat in clouds of noxious production fumes, and mining companies practiced only the slightest of safeguards against silica, coal, asbestos, and other dangerous dusts. Moreover, workers' homes provided little refuge. The crowded tenements of industrial cities—whether in the US Midwest or the German Ruhr-Westphalia—became breeding grounds for infectious diseases that respected no class lines even as they struck hardest at the poor, overworked, and undernourished working class. Together the new industries caused an overall decline in ambient air quality that decimated human health with pulmonary diseases, pulmonary fibrosis, asthma, and bronchitis.

The punishing industrial working conditions strengthened the socialist movements that had been active in Germany since the 1860s. Most prominent among these was the Socialist Workers' Party (Sozialistische Arbeiterpartei Deutschlands) that would in 1890 become the SPD, which exists to the present day. Workers' unions also experienced fantastic rises in membership, growing from 280,000 in 1890 to 680,000 in 1900.[15] Although ruled by an emperor (kaiser) from 1871 to 1918, Germany was hardly an absolute monarchy in the mold of the early kingdoms of France or even the contemporaneous czar of Russia. Nearly all men could vote for representatives to a federal legislature (Reichstag) that met in Berlin and played a significant if limited governing role. To be sure, Kaiser Wilhelm's chief government minister, Otto von Bismarck, as representative of the crown, held vast privileges, yet the elected SPD members of the Reichstag were not without freedoms to represent their working-class constituencies. In short, Germany's Second Reich, led by Wilhelm II (1871–1918), was not the totalitarian Third Reich led by Adolf Hitler between 1933 and 1945, under which leftists and union leaders were beaten into submission, imprisoned, or killed. However, even if Wilhelm was no Hitler, he nevertheless viewed socialism as an existential threat to the imperial German state. In response, he and Bismarck crafted two responses to undercut the growing power of the socialists and their support from industrial workers.

The first were the "antisocialist laws." These severely restricted SPD meetings of any kind, outlawed many trade unions, and banned socialist newspapers. The restrictions remained in place from 1878 to 1890. Bismarck justified the crackdown by falsely tying two assassination attempts on the kaiser to the socialist movement. In response, the socialists took their meetings underground, and socialist members of the Reichstag used their privileges as legislators to distribute their speeches, which essentially replaced the party's and union's banned newspapers. Given these countertactics, combined with the continuing deterioration of industrial working conditions, the leftist electorate continued to grow. Bismarck responded in a novel way: he sought to co-opt the SPD and its union allies through the creation of social insurance that protected workers against the risks of accidents, illness, and old age.

Existing institutions that cared for injured, sick, and elderly people were failing to meet the growing demand for their services in the new industrial cities. Protestant and Catholic charities were overwhelmed; trade union and guild sickness funds were chronically underfunded; and employer-based protections, though sometimes sufficient locally, were available only to workers at the largest firms.[16] Bismarck made the case to his conservative allies that repressive measures alone could not defeat socialism. The antisocialist laws, he said, had to be accompanied by positive measures of "moderate, reasonable state socialism."[17] Bismarck believed that if the monarchy could demonstrate its power to make workers more secure against ill health, accidents, and old age, industrial production could proceed unhindered by labor unrest and many workers would abandon socialism and vote for conservatives. As part of this strategy, he asked for government subsidies to pay for his social insurance plan. Indeed, Bismarck did not want employer or worker contributions to fund the new social safety net. The imperial state, he insisted, must be seen as the foremost benefactor of workers' entitlements to better health and improved well-being, so that the crown could reap the reward. Yet such a strategy could only work if Bismarck persuaded his fellow conservatives to approve a massive government expansion into the social realm. It also depended on compelling high levels of participation from industrial workers, many of whom were SPD members. The greater the number of participants, the lower the cost, because the risks of accident, illness, and old age would be spread across a large swath of the population.

Let us pause here to appreciate the scale of Bismarck's endeavor, however cunning its political motivations. At a time when the governments of other industrializing nations could only conceive of marginally effective child-labor laws and subsidies for private charities, Bismarck was insisting that the government alone should essentially finance the social needs of the entire industrial working class. Indeed, he believed that any requirement that workers contribute to the new safety net would erode their allegiance to the German state.[18] He wanted to completely efface the need for church-sponsored and especially worker-controlled social protections.

Not surprisingly, many of Germany's leading industrialists and free-market advocates bristled at Bismarck's suggestion that what was needed was "state socialism," a term that he openly embraced. They called his plans anti-market, patriarchal, and incompatible with the principles of progress and freedom.[19] One conservative leader remarked that Bismarck's proposal represented "the direct path to Communism."[20] Yet Bismarck refused to back down. "Many measures we have taken are socialist," he said, "and as it is, the state and our Reich will have to get used to a little more Socialism."[21] Despite criticisms from Bismarck's fellow conservatives, most of the country's industrial leaders eventually supported Bismarck's reforms if only because they could suggest no better answer to the increasingly militant working class. They wanted above all to preserve their power, which arose directly from their control over production and the capitalist economy. In the words of one industrialist who converted to Bismarck's cause, "The State must intervene to prevent further ruination, so that the stream of pauperism, growing incessantly, does not disastrously deluge the precious pastures of the fatherland."[22]

By the 1890s, Germany's capitalist elite had come to support reforms that offered stability during a turbulent period of social and economic transformation brought about by industrialization. They understood that the manufacturing sector could not be efficient without worker productivity. The philosophy of productivism drove a reconciliation between the conservative imperial state, which was under threat from both a potent socialist movement and an industrial elite who sought, above all, to avoid labor unrest in order to maintain production. Now it was the socialist leaders' turn to perceive an existential threat.

One of their founding leaders, Ferdinand Lassalle, called Bismarck's social insurance proposal "an attempt to open the valves in time to preempt an explosion [of socialist revolution]" and "to separate the working class from its leadership."[23] But absent a socialist majority in the Reichstag and no leftist voices in the throne room, the socialists could do little, at least in the beginning, to stop conservatives from co-opting a leftist program of worker protections and benefits. Pushed by Bismarck, the conservative majority in the Reichstag approved three waves of social legislation: illness insurance in 1883, accident insurance in 1884, and disability and pension provisions in 1889.

Bismarckian Social Insurance Laws

German workers had been cooperating to protect themselves against the risk of illness since the previous century and well before in some sectors. Guilds, fraternities, miners' associations, and factory unions had together succeeded in covering about one-quarter of the German working population. Yet even this limited success had been overwhelmed by the rapid growth of an industrial working class whose long shifts, dangerous work-places, poor diet, and unsanitary living environments produced sickness on a mass scale in German cities. Medical care, albeit cheap by modern standards, was relatively ineffective. In fact, prior to the mid-twentieth century, workers feared far more the loss of wages that resulted from the inability to work due to illness than the cost of medical care to treat the illness. Therefore, any illness insurance of the day that was worthy of its name had to include serious provisions for the replacement of wages during a worker's absence from work and convalescence. Bismarck's illness insurance met this expectation.

In addition to full coverage of physician fees and medications, Germany's 1883 illness insurance law provided up to thirteen weeks of sick pay equal to half the worker's wages, beginning on the third day of an illness or work injury–related absence. Prenatal women and new mothers could take four weeks of sick pay to give birth and to care for a new-born.[24] Moreover, medical coverage extended to injuries that occurred in the workplace. However, to Bismarck's chagrin, funding for these benefits relied on payroll deductions rather than general taxation. Workers paid two-thirds of the cost of their illness insurance and their employers paid one-third.[25] To provide medical services, the new illness insurance adopted a capitated reimbursement scheme similar to previous physician agreements with fraternities and unions where no fees were collected at the point of service. By 1900, illness insurance coverage had been extended well beyond the industrial working class and their family members; fully 62 percent of the population benefited from the new law. In 1903, the sick-pay period was doubled from thirteen to twenty-six weeks. And payments to doctors proved sufficiently generous so that by 1914 virtually all German ambulatory care physicians had signed up with their local district illness funds in order to care for the socially insured.

By the 1910s, German illness insurance was benefiting from what insurance experts call a "virtuous cycle." Its solid protection against the risk of illness meant that a growing number of workers wanted social insurance to be expanded to their professional classification, be it inland steam navigation or commerce or agriculture. As the group of beneficiaries became more varied and included more healthy, young participants, the more financially sound the illness insurance funds became, which permitted further improvements in benefits, thereby attracting greater interest from even more workers who were still outside the system, leading to another "virtuous cycle" of expansion. Bismarck's illness insurance successfully transformed Germany's health care system within twenty years, and it influenced those of neighboring countries, especially France where the German success could not be ignored.[26] In contrast, the accident insurance and pension laws of 1884 and 1889 were not destined for the same popularity, but they nevertheless proved foundational to the health of German workers and the productivity of the German economy.

Bismarck's 1884 workplace accident insurance law tackled early a problem faced by all industrializing societies of the time: when the all-too-common workplace accident struck, who should pay for a worker's medical fees, lost work time, and disability or death benefits? For decades, employers had insisted that the costs had to be borne by the party at fault, by which they usually meant the individual worker. But the blistering pace of plant machinery and the presence of dangerous materials left workers little margin for error. Because of mandatory long shifts, fatigued machine operators inevitably made mistakes, sometimes fatal, affecting themselves or their coworkers. Prior to 1884, when a worker's error resulted in serious injury or death, the employer bore no responsibility. Bismarck's accident insurance dispensed with fault as a determining factor in damage awards. Instead the law required employers to create insurance funds to pay for the costs of accidents on a no-fault basis.[27] As we will see, the United States would eventually implement a poor replica of this approach some twenty years later.

The final leg of Bismarck's social insurance triad concerned old age. The widespread adherence to productivism's normalization of wage labor could only be maintained if workers were promised a modicum of relief when their bodies could no longer work due to natural causes. The old-age insurance law of 1889 provided a small pension to workers who reached the age of seventy. But the pension law immediately fell afoul with workers. Its modest payments failed to constitute a livable wage-replacement, a disappointing outcome for a system into which workers paid in equal measure alongside their employers and the state. Worse, between 1900 and 1910 only 27 percent of men lived to see their seventieth birthday. Most therefore never saw the payment of their pension. An amendment to the law eventually allowed family members of a deceased worker to collect a portion of the pension, but it included restrictions on widows who remained gainfully employed.[28] Of greater importance to the program's eventual popularity was a 1916 amendment that lowered the age of retirement to sixty-five. Sixty-five thus became a standard retirement age for private and public pension systems across Europe and in many American states in the 1920s. President Franklin Roosevelt also adopted sixty-five as the normal retirement age for the 1935 Social Security Act.

Let us now return to how Bismarck's grand scheme to undercut his socialist rivals actually worked out. Socialists had been horrified by the advent of the social insurance laws of the 1880s, fearing they would undercut the appeal of unions and the SPD to workers. However, as the decades passed, it became clear that Bismarck's failure to convince his conservative allies to have the state pay for the new entitlements presented an extraordinary political boon for the socialists. Because workers paid two-thirds of the cost of the new illness insurance and half of the cost of the new pension program, conservatives were forced to concede that worker representatives, hence SPD leaders, should play an important role in the administration of social insurance. In short, absent the "state socialism" that Bismarck had failed to achieve, "social democracy" could develop.

The emergence of social democracy also stemmed from a mellowing of Germany's socialist movement. Earlier, in 1892, the SPD had announced, "Social Democracy is by its nature revolutionary, State Socialism is conservative. Social Democracy and State Socialism are irreconcilable opposites."[29] But by the early 1900s, the SPD had shifted its emphasis from revolution to evolution. Socialist leaders were now effective administrators of the German social insurance system, occupying powerful public roles that had previously been denied leaders from the political left. Moreover, the social insurance committees that administered the new benefits brought together workers, managers, leaders of employer associations, and trade unions, as well as factory inspectors. By the mid-twentieth century these committees would embody the "social partnership" that proved fundamental to the success of the modern German economy and the health of the nation.[30]

The American Workplace, 1880–1920

American factories, mines, and railways were even more dangerous than their European counterparts in the late nineteenth century. For example, approximately seventeen thousand US train crew members suffered serious injury every year, some 10 percent of the nationwide total of railway workers.[31] American railroads exhibited five times the accident rate of German or British railways. Fatal accidents in US coal mines were twice the rate of British coal mines and half again as much as their German counterparts. Despite these conditions, the *Wall Street Journal* opined in 1910, "Too much safety appliance robs the . . . employee of a responsibility which he ought to learn to bear."[32] Yet such a view increasingly fell on deaf ears as muckraking journalists, union leaders, and reformers refused to ignore developments in Germany and elsewhere in Europe where more health-conscious employers were simultaneously improving working conditions and productivity.

Few were more aware of the potential of European-style reforms to improve the health of American workers than activists in the Progressive movement. They are perhaps best known for their successful legislative initiatives to protect the food supply, namely the Pure Food and Drug Act and the Meat Inspection Act, both signed into law in 1906. Progressives recognized that the industrialization of the US economy had brought about such an unprecedented concentration of economic and political power that it enabled employers to disregard consumer, child, and worker safety. Hence, "trust busting," the breaking up of large commercial and industrial combines and monopolies, became intrinsic to the Progressive program. Virtually all of the Progressives, especially President Theodore Roosevelt, a Republican, and President Woodrow Wilson, a Democrat, justified their dismantling of trusts as a way to restore faith in (and the possibility of) small business entrepreneurship.

Unlike socialism, Progressivism's heritage can be traced to nineteenth-century laissez-faire theorists who believed fervently in the opportunities provided by open markets and democratic politics. Despite Progressives' belief in markets, their assessment of the early twentieth-century United States led them to believe that market opportunities had been exploited by a small number of economic titans, "robber barons," whose power had corrupted political life and threatened the very fabric of American democracy. Thus, Progressives marshaled the power of the government, through state ballot initiatives and legislation, the courts, and federal regulation, in an attempt to restore opportunity, equality, and justice, all of which they saw as necessary to ensure the progress of American civilization.[33]

Yet Progressive reformers faced an uphill battle and ultimately fell short of what the Germans had accomplished decades before. Two factors—one institutional, the second economic and demographic—are primarily responsible for the divergent outcomes in the United States and Germany. First, the Progressives lacked the levers of power that Bismarck and Kaiser Wilhelm enjoyed. Although these German leaders faced opposition from conservative industrialists who hewed closely to free-market principles, the monarchical nature of the Second Reich gave the German state tremendous power to implement reforms. Second, despite continued opposition from free-market conservatives, a critical mass of German leaders—from the monarchical right to the socialist left—agreed that social policies that protected workers' health could best ensure overall economic prosperity and growth. In contrast to the United States, where in-migration was strong, German industrialists and political leaders understood that the nation could not afford to treat its labor force as an expendable asset. Its health had to be preserved if productivity, political stability, and economic growth were to be sustained.

Germany's population grew substantially between 1871 and 1911, from 41,000,000 to 65,300,000, outdistancing growth rates in France and most other European countries.[34] Yet even this relatively rapid growth rate barely kept pace with the demand for workers from Germany's booming industrial sector. Meanwhile, during the same period, the US population grew from a lower base of 38,500,000 in 1870 to a total population of 92,200,000 in 1911, nearly thirty million greater than Germany's.[35] Moreover, a substantial portion of the US increase owed to in-migration, and many of the immigrants settled in the growing industrial centers of their new homeland, setting up a competition between themselves for relatively well-paid manufacturing jobs. As historian Christopher Sellers observes, "If native workers refused to risk bodily damage for daily income, the new arrivals often proved more willing, and the resultant competition for jobs gave American employers more leverage than their German and English counterparts to allow hazardous conditions to persist."[36] Under such circumstances, the Progressives were denied the unified working-class constituency that German socialist leaders enjoyed, which made health-promoting reforms more difficult to achieve.

It might appear that American reformers made up lost ground to Germany on accident and disability protections, known as workers' compensation.

Legislation in state after state in the early 1900s quickly settled the contentious issue of payments to workers who were injured or killed on the job. As late as 1897, most US observers had deemed workers' compensation insurance as "too radical to pass."[37] But, less than a decade later, President Theodore Roosevelt squirmed at the thought that Germany had protected its workforce through compulsory workers' compensation. Roosevelt admitted in 1908, "It is humiliating that at European international congresses on [workplace] accidents the United States should be singled out as the most belated among nations in respect of employers' liability legislation,"[38] The president's admission brought the full weight of the Republican Party to bear on the problem, but in the end the US solution only faintly resembled the German law that it was supposed to emulate.

New York passed the nation's first workers' compensation legislation in 1910; twenty-one states had followed by 1913, and a total of thirty-six states had passed comparable legislation by 1920. As noted in chapter 1, the reigning interpretation of the US Constitution did not permit federal legislation to take precedence over state laws. Therefore, the state reforms varied widely in their benefits and quality of protections. Even today, in Mississippi an employer can legally terminate an employee for exercising one's rights under the state's workers' compensation law.[39] Equally disappointing, many states allowed the participation of insurers who showed little interest in the prevention of workplace accidents in the first place. Bismarck's legislation forced German employers into special mutual insurance companies, governed by regulations that required them to take an active role in the prevention of workplace accidents. In the United States, by 1919, when the states completed adoption of their respective workers' compensation laws, fully 60 percent of the coverage had been handed to commercial insurers, 22 percent to state funds, and 18 percent to employer mutual funds. Experience showed that commercial insurers were far more willing to expend resources to fight claimant challenges to their policies in court than to invest in accident reduction measures at the workplace.[40]

As the effects of the new laws played out, it became clear that US employers had succeeded in limiting their liability while workers' access to on-the-job injury benefits had not improved by the same proportion, nor were the costs borne equitably across the labor force. Under all the US state laws, employers paid the full cost of no-fault insurance; in return, workers agreed that their payment for damages could not exceed insurance coverage levels. Yet only unionized workers succeeded in preventing employers from recouping their workers' compensation insurance premiums by lowering wages. Industrial union leaders understood that even if they could win some cases in court, in many cases they could not. They therefore accepted the new law. But nonunion workers who lacked the bargaining power of their unionized compatriots ended up paying their employers' insurance premiums through wage offsets, and they were prevented from bringing suit for accidents. They were not the only losers. Heeding the wishes of the farm lobby (and unopposed by the industrial union leaders), state legislators across the nation banned their agricultural and domestic workers, many of whom were African American (in the Southeast) and Hispanics (in the Southwest and West) from coverage under the new workers' compensation laws. Indeed, even today, sixteen states do not require agricultural employers to purchase workers' compensation insurance for seasonal employees, which can make up the bulk of the annual payroll for many farm operations.[41]

The US solution to workplace accidents settled the question of who is liable for work injuries but, in comparison to German law, failed to improve workplace safety to the same extent. Germany's accident insurance law concerned itself directly with the promotion of worker health alongside accident liability. As we saw earlier, the 1884 German workplace accident insurance law provided *supplementary* coverage to the 1883 illness insurance law, which already paid for worker injuries and maladies regardless of their origins in the workplace. Only after the employee had exhausted illness insurance benefits did workers' compensation take over. Therefore, in order to match German reforms in favor of worker health, US reformers would have had to achieve, in all the states, compulsory workers' compensation insurance that not only settled the issue of who paid but also the improvement in workplace safety. In addition, US reformers would have had to achieve passage of health insurance that included wage-replacement stipends, maternity leave, and medical care coverage. Indeed, a Progressive lobbying organization, the American Association for Labor Legislation (AALL), set out to achieve these very goals in the 1910s.

AALL leaders saw themselves as comprising "a disinterested party mediating between the two poles of capital and labor," a sort of think tank without a financial stake in the legislation it proposed. Before advocating for illness insurance, the AALL had taken the lead in several occupational health issues. One of its main investigators, the physician Alice Hamilton, emerged as the nation's foremost authority on occupational toxic disorders and is now considered the US founder of industrial medicine. Hamilton and the AALL succeeded in improving occupational health on several fronts by producing irrefutable epidemiological evidence that workers were being poisoned by carbon monoxide, mercury, and phosphorous. Indeed, the AALL successfully pressured Congress to ban the use of white phosphorous in manufacturing, which saved countless workers from a debilitating condition known as "phossy jaw." Drawn almost exclusively from academia—Hamilton was assistant professor of industrial medicine at Harvard—the AALL excelled at producing well-researched studies and policy papers that informed the drafting of legislation. Yet the forces arrayed against the AALL in the phosphorus case, mostly match manufacturers, were relatively small and easily tagged as self-interested. The battle for health insurance was larger and more complex.[42]

The AALL called their initiative "health insurance" rather than translating directly from the German to obtain "illness insurance." But their proposal bore a strong resemblance to Bismarck's 1883 law. Notably, the AALL bill benefited the mostly white male industrial working class whose labor was governed by wage contracts. Thus, like the workers' compensation laws, their proposed reform would exclude agricultural laborers in the Southeast, Southwest, and West. For workers who could participate, the bill offered substantial benefits in exchange for light premiums: 1.6 percent of wages. Employers would contribute the same, while the state paid 0.8 percent to create total revenues of 4 percent of wages. Like the German system, the draft bill envisioned local insurance funds as the "normal carrier." Payment for services would pass through the insurer to medical providers under a negotiated fee schedule or on a capitated basis. Alternatively, a local insurance fund might employ salaried physicians whom insured persons would have "reasonable free choice" selecting.[43] Also similar to the German system, wage replacement stipends covered approximately two-thirds of base pay for twenty-six weeks as well as maternity benefits for women.

The AALL plan found numerous supporters, especially in states where the Progressive movement was already strong. "Many wage earners, too proud to ask for charity treatment, get either no treatment at all, treatment too long delayed, or treatment of dubious value," stated the US Public Health Service in a 1916 pamphlet. It continued: "According to the experience in other countries as well as in the United States, private and commercial health insurance has failed to afford the relief and lighten the burden in the case of workers who stand in the greatest need."[44] In January 1917, a California state commission unanimously recommended the AALL draft bill to the state's legislature, nearly without change. Its findings underlined the political salience of government programs in favor of workers' health security. The commission noted, "The present *laissez-faire* method of ignoring the great problem of illness among wage-earning families until actual destitution demands public attention, [and it] is socially wasteful in the extreme."[45]

When US mobilization for the First World War in 1917 exposed high rates of poor health and disability among recruits, far higher than expected, the AALL quickly cast compulsory health insurance as a way to repair a dangerous chink in the nation's armor—its young fighting men. The Massachusetts Insurance Commission unabashedly explored the tension between individual liberty and the common good, a tension that members found comparable to the debate over the AALL bill. Commissioners conceded that it was "natural" to view compulsory health insurance as "an un-American infringement of the principle of personal liberty." But they likened health insurance to one of the few issues where the need for compulsion was generally agreed on: national defense. "Every male citizen in Massachusetts between certain ages is by law a member of its militia. . . . Let it once be recognized clearly that every citizen has a duty to prepare himself to meet the hazards of life such as sickness, unemployment, and dependent old-age."[46] That a legislative proposal on health insurance could induce such far-reaching arguments indicates how close it cut to the nerve of contested American values.

In April 1919, the New York State Senate, by a vote of thirty to twenty, approved the AALL's health insurance bill, but this was the first and last legislative body to approve the measure. Due in large part to a single recalcitrant committee chairman (and manufacturer), Thaddeus Sweet, the bill never reached the New York Assembly floor. Indeed, in state after state, Progressives were repeatedly disappointed. In California, an amended AALL proposal enjoyed the support of the state's insurance commission and Governor Hiram Johnson, who had been Theodore Roosevelt's running mate on the Progressive Party's presidential ticket in 1912. In true Progressive fashion, though, the California legislature submitted the measure to voters in a referendum. In response, the state's physicians created the California League for the Conservation of Public Health, whose sole purpose was to defeat the public health insurance proposal. On Election Day in November 1918, Californians trounced the measure, 63 percent to 37 percent.[47] In Illinois, Pennsylvania, Wisconsin, and Massachusetts—all states that the AALL had targeted for early approval—legislative efforts failed. Early momentum of public health insurance had withered in the face of public and private lobbying campaigns by insurers, physicians, employers, and their allies. Equally damaging, the head of American Federation of Labor (AFL), Samuel Gompers, spoke in ambivalent terms about the bill, which permitted critics to accuse the AALL of not really speaking for workers at all. Like many industrial union leaders to follow, Gompers believed that unions could negotiate a better deal on health coverage at the collective bargaining table. That may have been the case in the short term, but since its inception the AFL had belittled and excluded from its ranks both unskilled workers and immigrants. This tactic provided short-term gains for the mostly white skilled working men of the AFL, but it greatly weakened the US labor movement, whose power to protect workers from the risk of illness would ultimately rely on their solidarity regardless of skill, ethnicity, race, or gender.

In 1921, AALL head John Andrews announced that the leadership had "decided to await a more favorable time before again devoting so important a part of its modest resources to [the health insurance] campaign."[48] Prominent supporters of the AALL, including the New York Federation of Labor and the Women's Joint Legislative Conference of New York, also dropped public health insurance from their agendas. America's first battle to extend health insurance to working families was over.

Germany, 1919–1945

Germany's Second Reich failed to survive the nation's defeat in the First World War (1914–18). The war killed two million of the country's soldiers, four million more were severely wounded, and many were permanently disabled. On the home front, a British naval blockade forced severe food rationing throughout the country by April 1915. Food riots became common in large cities, and the government ordered that soup kitchens be established in all towns greater than ten thousand inhabitants so that residents could get at least one meal per day. Upon the armistice of November 1918, the humiliated Kaiser Wilhelm fled to neutral Holland. The socialist-led German republic that succeeded Wilhelm's rule was, from the beginning, dependent on social services to defuse domestic conflict. Indeed, the Weimar Republic—so-called because the National Assembly that drafted its constitution avoided a riotous Berlin in favor of the small provincial city of Weimar—became synonymous with reform and social democracy.[49]

The popular social insurance system that the new republic inherited from the Second Reich proved its most important institution in the struggle to maintain domestic peace. With right-wing militias already on the rise in the early 1920s—Adolf Hitler's first attempt at power came in 1923—the SPD moved quickly to bolster support from its working-class base. The government expanded accident insurance to include travel to and from work. It allocated new resources to medical services, increasing the number of doctors per capita in order to improve access to care. It also increased research funding, especially into the diagnosis of occupational diseases and therapies. Under the Weimar Republic, Germany became the first nation to officially recognize that radon caused uranium miners' lung cancer and began paying compensation to afflicted workers in the late 1920s. (US uranium miners would have to wait until 1991 for similar recognition and compensation.)[50] Weimar leaders also enforced constitutional measures that supported union participation and collective bargaining so that by 1922 nearly eleven thousand contracts applied to 890,000 businesses, representing 14,100,000 employees or 75 percent of the German labor force.[51] In contrast, US labor union membership remained below 10 percent until the 1935 Wagner Act provided legal protections for workers to organize, bargain collectively for wages and working conditions, and strike.[52]

Weimar leaders also scrambled to increase employment, both to serve their working-class constituency and to decrease the number of involuntarily idle men who could more easily be radicalized by the fledgling Nazi and other right-wing nationalist groups. The government established special labor courts and mediation procedures, making it harder for industrialists to shut down factories or summarily dismiss individual workers. It instituted job placement services and compulsory preferential hiring and retention protocols for veterans, who made up approximately half of all men in the labor force. Another key reform, whose significance cannot be overstated due to its eventual effect on worker health, was the 1920 creation of "works councils" in all enterprises with more than twenty employees. The law charged the new works councils, which were composed of workers and management "on an equal footing," with supporting "enterprise management with advice, in order thereby to ensure . . . the highest possible level of economic performance" and "concord among the workers and the employers."[53]

The Weimar labor reforms represented a strong social democratic agenda, but they retained the productivist goals of the earlier Bismarckian era that sought to protect the health of German workers to ensure worker productivity. This duality of purpose is apparent in the Weimar Constitution itself. Article 162 pledges that the state will "guarantee the rights of workers . . . [and] social rights for humanity's working class." Yet this constitutional commitment to protect the working class from an overbearing bourgeoisie is immediately followed by a productivist imperative of equal constitutional weight: "Notwithstanding his personal liberty, every German is obliged to invest his intellectual and physical energy in such a way as necessary for public benefit."[54] Throughout the 1920s, Weimar struggled to balance the competing claims of the workers and their unions, on the one hand, and the capital-owning classes, on the other, a struggle that was upended by the Depression of the 1930s. Business failures and mass unemployment overwhelmed Weimar's labor courts as the center of German politics evaporated. Voters lost faith in the SPD's centerleft social democracy. They either moved to the far right, especially to the Nazi Party, or to the far left, notably to the surging German Communist Party (KPD), enamored by leaders who promised to restore the economy and the nation.

In the 1930 elections, the communists' share of the Reichstag rose by 54 seats (of 577 total). Even more dramatic, though, was the rise of the National Socialist German Workers Party (NSDAP), commonly known as the Nazis, which added 95 members to its caucus in the Reichstag. Although Adolf Hitler lost his presidential bid in 1932 to the incumbent

Paul von Hindenburg, Hindenburg recognized the growing strength of the Nazis in 1933 by appointing Hitler to serve as chancellor and thereby manage day-to-day government operations and policies. Aided by a fire in the Reichstag, which Hitler blamed on leftist politicians, and Hindenburg's subsequent suspension of many civil liberties, the Nazis were able to dismantle the Weimar Republic through co-optation, intimidation, and violence. When Hindenburg died in office in 1934, Hitler combined the offices of the president and chancellor into a new position of leader and state chancellor (*Führer und Reichskanzler*) and assumed it himself. The new Nazi state banned the SPD, the KPD, and all independent worker unions, forcing their leaders to flee abroad in order to avoid arrest. The SPD thus lost all influence over the social insurance funds, which they had cultivated for decades.

In order to mollify German workers, most of whom had been members of the now-banned political parties and unions, the Nazis pursued a dual approach of inducement and coercion. They continued the expansion of job classifications that were covered by social insurance.[55] The regime also launched a series of jobs programs aimed at infrastructure, including a rapid acceleration of freeway (*Autobahn*) construction, which had been originally conceived by Weimar officials. The Nazis created a state-controlled leisure-time organization, Strength through Joy (*Kraft durch Freude*), that subsidized sporting clubs, concerts, plays, movies, and holiday travel for workers.[56] They launched a program to produce an affordable automobile—the *Volks-Wagen* (people's car)—for the working class. However, in order to pay for the design and production costs of the new car, the Nazis raided the assets of the state-controlled workers' union. Even then, very few of the new cars saw the light of day before production was suspended at the time of Germany's invasion of Poland in 1939. A similar fate befell Nazi infrastructural projects and the Strength through Joy program.[57] A notable exception was the National Socialist People's Welfare program (*Nationalsozialistische Volkswohlfahrt*). Through it the Nazi state seized control of most existing social welfare and charity programs, whether religious or secular, harnessing them to fulfill their goal of a healthful, sanitary utopia. The new Germany, the Nazis insisted, would eschew class distinctions. Instead, eugenics would inform a systematic exclusion and ultimately the murder of all who were deemed a threat to the well-being of a racially pure and unified people's community (*Volksgemeinschaft*).[58]

As under the Second Reich and the Weimar Republic, we see productivism as a driving force in the protection of worker health and safety in Nazi Germany. Workers were still protected from the dangerous environments inherent to modern industry so as to ensure their productivity. Yet in the Nazi version there existed no countervailing power to protect individual workers or minorities the regime identified as enemies of the nation. What unfolded next is surely the most barbarous paradox in the history of occupational safety. Workers who qualified as members of the national community (*Volksgemeinschaft*) benefited from the world's best health and safety research, toxic-substance mitigation apparatuses, and other protective technologies. Meanwhile, workers who were judged unfit to be members of the German nation, such as Jews, Sinti, Roma, communists, homosexuals, physically disabled people, and those with mental illness, were forced into slave-labor and extermination camps.

Within a year of the Nazi regime's accession to power in 1933, it moved aggressively to protect *Volksgemeinschaft* workers against one of the deadliest and most widespread occupational lung diseases: silicosis. Silicosis can result from relatively short-term exposure—one or two years—to quartz or silica dust. Mining, sandblasting, porcelain and brick manufacture, and iron foundries that use sand in casting molds commonly give rise to the hazards of silicosis. By April 1934, the Nazi quarrymen's union had established a new office to develop vacuum devices, hoods, filters, and ventilators for installation at the most affected worksites.[59] A poignant comparison between US employers' treatment of African American workers and those whom the Nazis considered racially deficient cannot be avoided here. In the very same year that Germany moved to protect its *Volksgemeinschaft* workers from silica dust, nearly five hundred African American miners were dying from exposure to exactly the same kind of dust while building the Hawk's Nest Tunnel in West Virginia. Court testimony subsequently revealed that the contractor, Union Carbide, had rejected slower wet-drilling techniques that would have greatly reduced the black workers' exposure to silica dust. Meanwhile, the all-white team of supervisors regularly wore protective breathing apparatuses but repeatedly denied the black miners' request for similar equipment.[60]

Nazi occupational health and safety efforts also proved effective at combating the threat of cancer. Historian Robert Proctor believes that this emphasis reflects the regime's racist ideology that viewed "Jews as tumors" and therefore "tumors as Jews."[61] Their top priorities included worker protections against asbestos-induced mesothelioma, a form of lung cancer, which the Nazi state recognized as a compensable occupational disease in 1943, making it the first nation to do so. The German Siemens corporation's newly developed electron microscope, which could detect the presence of extremely small fibers lodged in a worker's lung tissue, was harnessed to discern the etiology of asbestosis. Using specially developed pathological techniques and animal testing, German researchers moved quickly from clinical evidence drawn from very few human cases to directly implicate asbestos dust as the cause of asbestosis and mesothelioma.[62]

As the exigencies of war increased by 1942, the Nazi state's regard for occupational health waned, even for bona fide members of the *Volksgemeinschaft*. Workers were to be protected but only if such protections did not interfere with production schedules. In this way, the Nazi state abandoned the productivist agenda that had reigned since Bismarck's day and the Weimar Republic. No longer was the health and vitality of workers to be protected in order to safeguard long-term production and productivity. The short-term survival of the Nazi regime was all that mattered. Individual workers could be consumed in the same way their machines were overworked and discarded. Any worker illness that prevented productive presence at the workplace became dangerous, even potentially fatal. Individuals who could not contribute to the nation's war effort opened themselves to the charge that they had become extraneous to the nation and could be liquidated to preserve increasingly scarce food resources. To be sure, the plight of concentration camp laborers became incomparably worse as the prospects for German victory diminished.

Whether inside or outside the camps, elderly people became a preferred target for elimination. German Labor Front officials openly stated that the difference between the age of retirement and the age of death should be zero.[63] Clearly, the Nazis had lost all regard for Bismarck's third social insurance law of 1889 that guaranteed a pension at age sixty-five. To them, no life, no matter how productive in the past, could be allowed to burden the German nation from its supposed destiny of purity and domination. That the German Labor Front, which under the Third Reich had replaced the nation's once powerful workers' unions, could take such a position toward older workers is a testament to how thoroughly the Nazis had abandoned the long-term productivism of German industry in favor of a racial state bent on world supremacy.

Rebuilding German Productivism, 1945–1991

Only after the utter defeat of the Nazi regime and the total occupation of German territory could state and autonomous union leaders again collaborate in rebuilding a productivist agenda that embraced the health of workers. But within a few short years it became clear that that rebuilding would be quite different in the Soviet zone of occupation. The Allied Control Council, made up of members from Britain, France, the Soviet Union, and the United States, splintered. The American, British, and French representatives acted to encourage commercial and economic collaboration among the three western zones, including the introduction of a new common currency, the Deutsche Mark. In March 1948, Soviet member Vasily Sokolovsky walked out of an Allied Control Council meeting, never to return. A new state, the Germany Democratic Republic (GDR) was created the following year, led by the Socialist Unity Party of Germany (SED) and backed by the Soviet Union. With this merger of the interwar socialist and communist parties, one might have expected that Germany's pre–Nazi era social insurance and works councils would reemerge as a locus of autonomous working-class power in the new East Germany. Yet it quickly became clear that the communists, backed by the Soviet Occupation Authority, held the upper hand; the socialists proved ineffectual in steering GDR policy. While certain German workplace practices were respected, the SED secretary Walter Ulbricht asserted state control over social policy, including social insurance.

The East German government combined the separate social insurance funds that covered workplace accidents, disability, illness, and old age, and it proclaimed "the right to work" for all citizens. The promise of "jobs for all" cost the regime dearly in terms of economic efficiency but was never renounced. In fact, throughout its existence (1949–91) the GDR remained relatively productive and wealthy by east European standards, matching the growth rates and living standards of its master and protector, the USSR. Even West German observers of the GDR's health system gave it high marks for its emphasis on preventive services and coordination of care, both for ambulatory and acute-care patients. At the center of the GDR's health system stood a state-paid primary-care physician with broad powers to convoke specialty care providers. In 1953, a construction labor strike morphed into mass protests against the government and necessitated the deployment of Soviet troops to restore order. Afterward, the communists further expanded health and family benefits to bolster support for the regime.[64]

Taken in sum, though, East Germany failed to maintain and improve the health of its population at the same rate as its western neighbor, the Federal Republic of Germany (FRG), to which East German health outcomes were inescapably compared. Foreign actions played an important role in the tale of the two German states. Initially, the US and British governments plundered German patent and intellectual property in order to enrich their own national industries. Yet by 1947 these policies gave way to sustained cash and in-kind assistance under the US Marshall Plan that greatly aided West Germany's economic recovery. In contrast, the Soviet Union insisted on long-term war reparations from East Germany, especially in the form of capital equipment that the country badly needed to relaunch economic growth. Although not without its achievements, when compared to West Germany, the GDR entered a period of economic stagnation and a decline in the social determinants of health. Retirement pensions were notoriously low, never rising above 50 percent of the mean wage; the country's housing stock remained insufficient and dilapidated; and care for those with disabilities was chronically underfunded and its methods obsolete.

Even the aforementioned health care system ultimately could not maintain its effectiveness due to a physician shortage. When the government took full control of health care, it cut payments to private-practice physicians. This prompted a massive emigration of doctors to West Germany, which was easily accomplished prior to the GDR's closing of the inter-German border and the building of the Berlin Wall in the summer of 1961. Between 1946 and 1961, East Germany lost approximately seventy-five hundred physicians, about half of its medical corps, a disproportionately high share of whom were young practitioners.[65] As daily living conditions and health care access stagnated in East Germany, life expectancy in West Germany regained and then surpassed prewar levels. Indeed, by the 1980s, the amenable mortality rate in East Germany—deaths that could have been prevented through timely and effective health care—rose to 4.6 times that of West Germany. As early as 1965, East German leaders recognized their dilemma. They were far from achieving an "inviting example" for all Germans, which had been their hope immediately after the war. SED secretary Ulbricht admitted in an internal discussion, "We're pressed by the competition with West Germany. . . . We were saying just 10 years ago that we are superior, [but now] pensions, health insurance have reversed. West Germany is better, even in health insurance."[66] Amazingly, one aggrieved East German citizen claimed in a court petition regarding a disputed social benefit, "I'm worse off here than an unemployed person in the FRG [West Germany]." Despite his clear swipe at the regime, he won his case; the judge noted "grounds recognized" on the plaintiff's file.[67] Dire though the comparisons between East and West Germany may be, we must also remember that by the late 1980s West Germany had also surpassed the United States on many health outcomes, a phenomenon that continues in the present day.

A major causal factor in West Germany's health achievements can be attributed to what Germans still today call the "social market economy" (*soziale Marktwirtschaft*), which seeks to reconcile the workings of the market with the greater social good and individual needs. To be sure, the Socialist Party (SPD) left a political legacy from the nineteenth and early twentieth centuries on which the social market economy could be built. However, the economy's main architects after the Second World War hailed from the center-right Christian Democratic Union party (CDU), which brought together center-right anti-Nazi politicians who had survived from the interwar period. Foremost among them stood Konrad Adenauer, the Zentrum (Center) Party leader and mayor of Cologne who had been removed from office in 1933 and twice imprisoned by the Nazis. Equally important was Adenauer's minster of economics, Ludwig Erhard, who engineered West Germany's "economic miracle" (*Wirtschaftswunder*) of the 1950s and 1960s. Adenauer and Erhard, alongside the leaders of the West German states (*Länder*) drafted the Basic Law (*Grundgesetz*), which became the Federal Republic's de facto constitution after 1949. It bolstered many of the pro-health dimensions of the old interwar Weimar Constitution, including the notion of the "social state," which denotes the responsibility of the government and civil institutions to actively promote equity and health. Both the social market economy and the social state remain constitutive principles of the German polity today. From them, Germans derived the laws, institutions, and social policies that help to explain the comparatively strong health outcomes of their working-age population.[68] The FRG's various state constitutions likewise reflected this commitment. For example, that of Rhineland-Palatinate notes, "The organization of economic life must accord with the principles of social justice, with the goal of guaranteeing a dignified existence for all."[69]

West Germany also benefited from the renaissance of powerful trade and employees' unions and works councils, the latter of which were first created under the Weimar Republic in the 1920s. The Deutscher Gewerkschaftbund (DGB) emerged as the dominant union confederation; its member unions were present in most heavy industries, as well as retail, finance, and some public sectors.[70] The metalworkers' group, IG Metall, became the largest union of the DGB confederation and the single largest industrial union in Europe. It included the German auto and aircraft manufacturing sectors as well as chemical, steel, and associated industries. The power of IG Metall influenced worker compensation in other sectors, including non-union industries, driving wages higher as West Germany's economy boomed during the economic growth of the late 1950s and 1960s. Yet the power of unions to raise living standards and thus health outcomes is only part of the story.

German workers benefited from employee-run works councils and the new institutions of codetermination (*Mitbestimmung*) to build a "stakeholder society." It ensures that the fruits of productivism are shared more equitably in Germany than in the United States, and not only in terms of income distribution but also in terms of power within the workplace, a critical determinant of workers' health. German unions insist that a fair share of a firm's productivity gains flow to worker compensation. But in Germany there is an additional lever that employees have at their disposal: works councils. Whether they work on the shop floor or in offices, works councils provide employees greater control over their labor. Any firm with more than five employees may create a works council, which is composed of elected members. Council size rises with the number of workers. It might only possess one employee for a small company of less than twenty workers. But a corporation that employs thousands may possess a works council of several dozens to address its various sectors and workplace environments. Workers' codetermination powers in large firms also extend to the supervisory board. Employees may occupy one-third of the seats in companies between five hundred and two thousand workers and half of the board seats in companies with more than two thousand employees. Employees who sit on a firm's supervisory board or works council are paid to carry out their duties to improve productivity, working conditions, and employee health.

A works council's health and safety committee (*Arbeitsschutzausschuss*) plays an important role in the occupational environment of any firm. In contrast to the United States, where typically underfunded state and federal agencies regulate workplace safety from outside the company, German workers and employers collaborate in-house to fulfill this task. German state regulatory agencies need only resolve disputes.[71] But the health and safety committee provides only part of the health benefits bestowed on German workers. Works councils and codetermination ensure a measure of employee control over the firm's overall operations. For example, in retail establishments, the employer must collaborate with the works council when setting opening and closing hours, employee shifts, vacation-time rotations, the introduction of new technologies, and even personnel matters, such as disciplinary processes.[72] In short, German workers, regardless of whether their firm or sector is unionized, have more power than their US counterparts. And epidemiological studies have demonstrated important links between greater employee control over their work and improved health outcomes.[73]

United States, 1920–1991

The United States has never developed the kind of shared management practices that bolster German workers' health. Nor has the United States built a comprehensive social insurance system along German lines to cover workplace accidents, disability, old age, and health care. That said, some American firms learned early in the twentieth century that workplace safety could be enhanced by appointing workers to management-controlled accident-prevention teams. And, in 1930s, the United States made a large stride toward protecting its workers against destitution in old age.

The 1932 presidential contest between Democrat Franklin Roosevelt and Republican incumbent Herbert Hoover turned on the candidates' contrasting remedies for the Depression and social reform. The health of Americans per se was not on the ballot. The Democratic platform pledged federal aid for rural America and support for veterans' pensions, but it also promised a reduction in federal spending and a balanced budget. Plans to create German-style public health insurance was nowhere to be seen. Nonetheless, a general air of anxiety spread over Republican circles about the contours of Roosevelt's promised "New Deal." Indeed, immediately after the election, Hoover openly asked for assurances from the president-elect that he contemplated no radical measures. The deft Roosevelt responded reassuringly without being specific about his plans.

In this context, an editorial in the *Journal of the American Medical Association* came as a preemptive volley directed at possible New Deal health care initiatives. The AMA pronounced in 1932, "[The] alignment is clear—on the one side the forces representing the great foundations, public health officials and social theory—even socialism and communism—inciting to revolution; on the other side, the organized medical profession of this country urging an orderly evaluation guided by controlled experimentation which will observe principles that have been found through the centuries to be necessary to the sound practice of medicine."[74] The AMA's attempt to associate public health leaders and health care reformers with communist revolutionaries would not be its last.

Many opponents of the New Deal considered it un-American because of its expansion of federal power in the economy and society. In particular, reformers and public health professionals who had supported the Children's Bureau activities in the 1920s were subjected to a fierce barrage of ad hominem attacks throughout the 1930s and 1940s.[75] The composition of Roosevelt's Committee on Economic Security, which was charged with drafting the Social Security Act, made opponents of health reform especially anxious. Equally worrisome was the plight of their own camp. Commercial insurers who had funded an array of umbrella organizations in opposition to the earlier AALL public health insurance initiative had been debilitated by the Depression. Virtually all of them were either in or near bankruptcy, forcing their leaders to call upon Roosevelt, hat in hand. Roosevelt duly obliged them, authorizing federal government–backed loans by the Reconstruction Finance Corporation. However, once on the public dole, the once powerful commercial insurance lobby could do little more than whisper their alarm at the growing strength of the health care reform forces.[76]

Organized labor's position had also changed. During the AALL battle over public health insurance, the American Federation of Labor leader Samuel Gompers had opposed government intervention, arguing that workers' unions should seek independent solutions at the collective bargaining table. But William Green succeeded Gompers as head of the AFL in 1924, and Green adopted the opposite position on public health insurance. Green had cofounded the United Mine Workers, whose workplaces were infamous for their acute dangers to health. In recognition of labor's importance to the New Deal coalition and Green's support for social insurance, Roosevelt appointed him to the Committee on Economic Security, where he strenuously argued for the inclusion of public health coverage in the definition of "social security." The coalition that had defeated the AALL's campaign for public health insurance in 1920 had now been whittled to the AMA and employers. Yet even these well-respected lobbies appeared vulnerable in the tumult of the Depression.

In his 1933 inaugural address, Roosevelt spoke at length about the financial crisis that afflicted the nation, which is not surprising since so many Americans had lost their life savings in bank failures. But Roosevelt went well beyond promises to restore a crippled banking system. He scornfully attacked bankers for their "false leadership" and pledged to "apply social values" in a restoration of the country's banks. A major portion of the new president's speech was devoted to an attack on the hallowed professional sovereignty of bankers, justifying massive government intrusion to its core. Taking this along with Roosevelt's repeated recognition of the citizenry's "interdependence on each other; that we cannot merely take but we must give as well," AMA leaders had to assume that the president regarded doctors' professional sovereignty not as an inalterable truth but rather as contingent on the social needs of the nation.[77] Seen in this light and given the unmet health needs of the population, many AMA officials assumed that Roosevelt was preparing a renewed initiative for public health insurance.

In fact, White House staff were planning to include government-sponsored health insurance in the Social Security Act. But Labor Secretary Frances Perkins and Committee on Economic Security director Edwin Witte became anxious that a fight over health care could undermine their ability to get any social legislation through Congress. The White House had been receiving a steady stream of letters and telegrams from doctors who opposed any New Deal initiative on health care, the product of a nationwide campaign orchestrated by the AMA. Newspaper editorials also began to appear, bearing the same arguments as the doctors' letters. Despite the public campaign that had been opened against them, many in the White House insisted that a large portion of the medical profession would eventually support the inclusion of health insurance in the Social Security Act. Yet throughout the fall of 1934 the letters, telegrams, and newspaper editorials kept coming. Finally, in November, Perkins and Witte pulled the plug. They advised Roosevelt to drop health insurance from the Social Security Act for fear that it would jeopardize the entire bill, including the public pension program that Americans enjoy today. The sagacity of Perkins and Witte's advice soon became apparent in congressional hearings. Such a chorus of lawmakers spoke against public health insurance that even its mention as a topic of research had to be struck from Social Security in order for the bill to move forward.[78]

Roosevelt could only have been impressed by the AMA's show of force and the concomitant weakness of groups advocating for health insurance. The unions and farm bureaus failed to rally anywhere near a comparable display of congressional support. In contrast to compulsory pensions and unemployment insurance, public health insurance appeared to have lost the reform energy that it had enjoyed in the days of the AALL campaign two decades earlier.[79] Although Roosevelt never publicly conceded defeat on health care reform, he never again risked substantial political capital for its attainment.

The dilemma Roosevelt faced demonstrated again how racism shaped the US health system. Southern Democrats had benefited disproportionately from Roosevelt's 1932 Democratic landslide, and their leaders continued their ascension to the chairs of a congressional committee system that rewarded seniority. Publicly funded health insurance would have meant a substantial change to the health care delivery system in the Jim Crow South, where health care facilities for African Americans were separate and inferior (or, in some regions, nonexistent). The Democratic Party's southern wing mistrusted Roosevelt's massive expansion of federal executive power—power that Republican and Democratic conservatives alike viewed as a danger to states' rights. If Roosevelt pushed his southern Democratic colleagues too hard, he risked defections, which could have brought the New Deal and Roosevelt's own continued electoral success to a halt.[80] In addition, the AMA's impressive campaign against public health insurance fell on fertile ground. The AMA was a confederation of state medical societies and therefore well capable of cultivating regional leaders who could lobby their members of Congress in the local dialect. Their insistence that government-sponsored health insurance constituted a federal invasion of medical sovereignty and would crush the traditions of private-practice medicine possessed a poignant metaphor for southerners' bitter history with federal power. Unlike public health insurance, the Social Security Act's headline features—old age and unemployment insurance—possessed no comparably invasive features. Both employers and workers were asked to contribute on equal terms to a pension system that remained firmly linked to private labor markets, and business leaders supported it.[81]

Even so, southern legislators insisted on the exclusion of agricultural and domestic workers, whose ranks were filled with African Americans, from Social Security pensions. These same workers were also excluded from many other New Deal relief programs, including the National Recovery, Agricultural Adjustment, National Labor Relations, and Fair Labor Standards Acts. As a result, 90 percent of the African American labor force in the South did not benefit from most New Deal programs. As historian Colin Gordon explains, "[The] implications of the agricultural exclusion were also quite clearly specific to the South and Southwest—regions whose economies were dominated by agriculture, whose agricultural systems were peculiarly labor intensive, and whose agricultural labor markets were organized around low wages, tenancy, harsh legal controls, and violence."[82]

Roosevelt's Social Security Act became law in 1935. American political leaders could not again agree on major social reform legislation to promote health and welfare until the 1950s, when Social Security was finally extended to agricultural workers, the self-employed, and other sectors. The 1950s also saw the creation of Aid to the Permanently and Totally Disabled, a forerunner of Supplemental Security Income (SSI), an assistance program to help nonparticipants in Social Security, and Social Security Disability Income (SSDI), which extended support only to those workers who had made substantial contributions to Social Security. During its first ten years, only workers over age fifty were eligible for SSDI, no matter the nature or level of their incapacitation. Subsequently and unfortunately, both SSI and SSDI have been plagued by inconsistencies in eligibility across states and between administrative law judges who determine a disabled worker's eligibility for benefits.[83]

Most US employers joined physicians in opposing a German-style public health insurance system in the 1930s. But they were interested in improving workplace safety. As we saw earlier, workers' compensation insurance had been enacted by the states in the early decades of the century. C. W. Crownhart of the Wisconsin Industrial Commission summed up the circumstances well: "Since the Workman's Compensation Acts . . . more real safety work has been done in the United States than in any ten years preceding." Magnus Alexander of General Electric agreed: "Barring a few notable exceptions, employers . . . did not get very busy on . . . accident prevention and safeguarding until they were forced by legislation."[84] Workers' compensation legislation was far from the first safety law. Regulations that sought to avoid railway, factory, and mine accidents had been on the books for decades. But weak enforcement and their limited scope did little to decrease overall worker injuries and death, which is why, as described earlier, German accident rates in the same industries were so much lower. Economist Martin Aldrich explains that the employers' workplace safety movement only began in earnest when accidents could no longer be blamed on workers but were instead seen as the failure of management, which in turn, threatened the firm's bottom line.[85]

US Steel pioneered the American safety movement, beginning in 1908, and dozens of other large firms emulated its measures in succeeding decades. At the center of US Steel's approach stood the frontline workers. Their knowledge of the production process and its most hazardous aspects informed many of the firm's health and safety improvements. Yet because US employers were not compelled to grant their employees powers similar to those of German works councils, the American safety movement failed to achieve the same success. Nevertheless, US frontline workers and management together conducted educational campaigns that included posters and safety contests. Workers also collaborated with company engineers to produce a substantial research literature on accident rates and prevention techniques. It showed that the injury rate in US heavy industry (but not smaller firms) fell by approximately 50 percent between 1926 and 1945.[86]

Ultimately, voluntarism placed a limit on how far the US worker safety movement could go. The favorable cost-benefit analysis that drove the movement in heavy industry—steel, railroads, and chemicals—often failed to compute for small or even medium-sized firms where most Americans worked. And no matter the firm size, safety committees did not possess the power to prevail over management in the same way as the health committees of German works councils. Sometimes even insurance companies could not persuade employers to invest in safety apparatus. For example, in 1931, Liberty Mutual Insurance informed textile manufacturer Bancroft Mills that additional safeguards should be added to its production line and that such changes would lower Bancroft's workers' compensation insurance premiums. The company rejected the advice, saying that "neither the premium saving nor the hazard involved would justify making the required changes."[87] When health remained a fungible commodity, subject to the same financial calculations as capital equipment, raw materials, and other production inputs, worker health suffered. In Germany, the combination of an effective social insurance system and the authority of employee works councils balanced the distribution of power between labor and management in the interest of safety. Meanwhile US workers had to rely on state agencies to protect them from occupational hazards and to improve workplace health. Unfortunately, time and again, federal and state regulators proved incapable of providing such protections.

Indeed, one of the leading companies in the US worker-safety movement of the 1920s, DuPont Chemicals, was also one of the most reckless in regard to workers' health. This paradox is possible because firms that led the worker-safety movement concerned themselves primarily with accidents that resulted in immediate injuries and therefore productivity losses and higher workers' compensation insurance premiums. But they willfully neglected the dangers that exposure to toxic substances posed to their employees' long-term health. In the case of Dupont, production processes at its organic chemicals plant in Deepwater, New Jersey, exposed workers to benzidine and beta-naphthylamine (BNA) at a time when chemical manufacturers around the world knew them to be carcinogens. Indeed, Germany, also a leading producer of organic chemicals, had made diseases associated with exposure to benzidine and BNA, notably bladder cancer, compensable in 1925, following the publication of an International Labour Organisation (ILO) study that demonstrated their risks. But in the United States neither federal nor state workplace safety regulators adhered to the ILO recommendations concerning protective apparatuses.

Nor did they follow Germany's lead in recognizing employer liability for failing to protect workers. Equally troubling, internal documents reveal that DuPont managers were aware that workers were subject to "gross exposure" to benzidine and BNA beginning in 1919. Many of those workers presented with bladder cancer in the early 1930s. In 1947, the medical director admitted in a letter to one of the affected workers who was still alive, "The question of health control of employees in the manufacture of Beta Naphthylamine is indeed a grave one. As you know, we have manufactured Beta Naphthylamine for many years. Of the original group who began the production of this product, approximately 100% have developed tumors of the bladder." Acknowledging its dangers, all European producers banned manufacturing processes that employed BNA by 1955, and many did so as early as 1938. However, the United States allowed its use in manufacturing with virtually no protections for workers until the mid-1960s.[88]

Even when US government agencies were committed to reigning in employers' disregard for their workers' health, regulators could not prevail over the power of recalcitrant employers. In 1938, the US Public Health Service teamed up with state investigators to conduct an epidemiological study in three asbestos tile factories in North Carolina. When they arrived at the plants they learned that employers had adopted a scorched-earth response to their inquiry. They had terminated 150 workers whose length of tenure and jobs at the plants placed them at most risk. Investigators tracked down sixty-nine of the fired employees. Forty-three of them had asbestosis. Asbestos manufacturers subsequently launched a sophisticated campaign to cast doubt on the link between asbestosis, a debilitating disease in its own right, and mesothelioma. A German immigrant to the United States, the toxicologist Wilhelm Heuper, had identified a troubling correlation between asbestosis and mesothelioma in 1942. (Heuper would go on to head the National Cancer Institute's Environmental Cancer Section.) Based on evidence provided by the newly invented electron microscope, the Nazi regime made asbestosis and mesothelioma compensable occupational diseases. In 1949, the American Medical Association concurred with the German findings. But US government agencies refused to enact measures to protect the health of asbestos industry workers, whether or not they were directly involved in its manufacturing or its application in the building trades. Only after 1964, when the industry's propaganda war against scientific findings began to fall apart, did the United States finally enact the health protections that European workers had enjoyed for decades.[89] The impotence of the US Public Health Service and state agencies in protecting US worker health provides a striking contrast to the effective shop-floor institutions and government agencies in comparably industrialized nations in Europe. The founder of industrial medicine in the United States, Alice Hamilton, died at the age of 101 in 1970. Despite her longevity, she failed to witness the creation of a federal agency in the Department of Labor whose mission would be to safeguard worker health.

President Richard Nixon signed the Occupational Safety and Health Act (OSHA) in December 1970. Only seven years later, OSHA came under attack as part of a larger effort to deregulate US industry in the face of a stagnant economy. President Jimmy Carter advocated the adoption of economic incentives and voluntary measures in lieu of the legal enforcement of safety standards.[90] Another blow came in 1978 when the US Supreme Court ruled that OSHA inspectors would henceforth be required to obtain search warrants to inspect commercial buildings for occupational hazards. Previous OSHA rules allowed for an inspector to make unannounced inspections of commercial premises "during regular working hours and other reasonable times within reasonable limits and within a reasonable manner." But when an OSHA inspector arrived at Barlow Electrical and Plumbing in Pocatello, Idaho, in September 1975 to conduct a routine inspection, the owner, Ferroll G. Barlow, denied access to the premises based on grounds that the inspection would violate his protection from an unreasonable search guaranteed by the Constitution's Fourth Amendment. The US Supreme Court ruled in Barlow's favor. Again, as in the early decades of the twentieth century, the primacy of voluntary employer compliance emerged as critical to the case. Writing for the majority, Justice Byron R. White noted that "the great majority of businessmen can be expected in normal course to consent to inspection without warrant," and he asserted, "[OSHA] has not brought to this court's attention any widespread pattern of refusal." By this reasoning, White continued, "The advantage of surprise will not be lost if, after entry to an inspector is refused, an *ex parte* warrant can be obtained, facilitating the inspector's reappearance at the premises without further notice."[91] An *ex parte* warrant may be issued without the employer's knowledge. The Supreme Court's decision in the Barlow case, however, means that OSHA safety inspectors, who are members of the executive branch, may need the permission of another branch of government—the judiciary—to carry out routine duties, a hurdle usually only required of criminal law enforcement officers. As White noted in his majority opinion, the court preferred to rely on the voluntary cooperation of employers, which has continued to be historically congruent with the US approach to worker health since the late nineteenth century. Reliance on employers' voluntary compliance affects the overall safety of US workplaces. The difference between on-the-job fatality rates of American and German workers is stark. Germany's occupational fatality rate (deaths per hundred thousand workers per year) is 48 percent lower than that of the United States, a remarkable statistic in light of the fact that Germany's manufacturing sector, where many occupational hazards are concentrated, is double that of the United States as a percentage of the national economy.[92]

A growing body of evidence indicates that greater worker control creates feelings of mutual support and leads to better worker health outcomes and productivity. Since the 1970s, research conducted on both sides of the Atlantic has repeatedly demonstrated that greater worker influence over workplace practices, such as scheduling, the use of new technologies, and the measurement of individual productivity, reduces workers' risk of both direct and indirect physiological and psychological illnesses. Many dangerous chronic conditions and diseases, including hypertension, elevated serum cholesterol, coronary heart disease, cardiovascular ailments, and gastrointestinal illnesses, appear to be in part caused by insufficient worker power over their jobs. A modicum of worker control also appears to benefit employees' mental health and to bring about a decrease in individual behaviors that diminish health outcomes, including attempted suicide, drug- and alcohol-related illnesses, and self-reported anxiety and depression.[93] The use of contingent workers who often exhibit the least control over their workplace environments is more restricted in Germany than in the United States.[94] Indeed, the United States has witnessed a 36 percent rise in contingent workers since 2005. Forty percent of US workers now rely on unsecure employment in which power over their work, access to employer-sponsored health insurance, paid sick leave, and other benefits are substantially reduced in comparison to traditional employees.[95]

The evidence that demonstrates the causal link between improved worker control and better health outcomes raises the question of how to protect worker health in the face of growing global production supply chains. In order to meet the exigencies of competitive worldwide markets, managers often feel compelled to place their employees in demanding circumstances with little control over their work. German-style works councils appear to provide an answer to this apparent dilemma. For example, on the question of scheduling, studies demonstrate that nonstandard work hours (e.g., night, swing, and split shifts), which casual observers may assume are detrimental to health because they violate circadian rhythms, have only been found to be detrimental when also accompanied by insufficient worker control over scheduling.[96] Another study addressed the issue of job insecurity, an increasingly common phenomenon caused by the growth of contingent workers in the US and in Europe. The researchers concluded, "Organizations can temper the negative health effects of job insecurity by giving their workers more control over their work."[97] Even in an environment of heightened global competition and automation, German-style works councils and codetermination actually contribute to firm productivity and thereby facilitate the protection of high-level compensation at the collective bargaining table. As economists Joel Rogers and Wolfgang Streeck note, "Councils appear capable of making an *efficiency* contribution to the performance of advanced industrial democracies, improving both individual *firm productivity* and the *effectiveness of state regulation* (economic or social) of firms."[98]

The achievement of power-sharing in the workplace, so well represented by the institutions of works councils and codetermination, helps to explain why the health outcomes of Germany's working-age population have remained strong even as the proportion of the German labor force that belongs to a union has fallen, from approximately 40 percent to 20 percent since the Second World War.[99] Germany's stakeholder society, which bestows substantial health benefits on its working-age population, shows no comparable signs of going away. In contrast, US working-age adults have historically suffered from a relative absence of power in the workplace, a key social determinant of health, which may explain the relatively poor health outcomes of American working-age adults compared to their German counterparts.

Indeed, worker power may be the most important theme from our historical examination of the social determinants of health for working-age adults in Germany and the United States. Viewed broadly, it captures the contrasting manner with which the two nations have negotiated the fundamental tension between workers' strivings to protect themselves from the health risks of everyday life, on the one hand, and employers' insistence on productivity gains, on the other. We have seen that, during the last century and a half, workers and employers of both nations have embodied the tenets of productivism: the overarching belief that the principal goal of socioeconomic activity in a market economy is to seek productivity gains through innovation and individual initiative that will together result in rising economic output and prosperity. Yet German workers and employers have succeeded more consistently in the sharing of power over socioeconomic activity, which has ultimately proven more beneficial to worker health and productivity gains.

The most striking example is the comprehensive system of worker accident, disability, and health coverage whose origins in Germany date to the 1880s. The administration of German social insurance by the Socialist Party and union leaders during the early decades of the twentieth century is a testament to power sharing in the socioeconomic realm. So too is the powerful role of works councils in German firms of all sizes, an innovation that dates to the Weimar Republic of the 1920s. In fact, the German principle that employers and workers are partners at both the firm and national levels may prove to be as essential to workers' health as it is to the survival of market economies in the fast-moving and increasingly globalized world of the twenty-first century.

3

AFTER WORK IN THE UNITED STATES AND SWEDEN

The Swedes themselves are not entirely sure what they have done right.

—PAUL KRUGMAN, *THE GREAT UNRAVELING*

Uppsala, Sweden. I wake in an unfamiliar bedroom, flooded with sunlight. I had arrived from Paris in the wee hours, and my friend had insisted that I would be more comfortable lodging at her grandmother's house than at her own small apartment. Chatting voices now emanate from downstairs although I was told that Grandma lived alone. I dress and descend the stairs to meet her. She is eighty years old, slim, and sharp of mind but unsteady on her feet. Attending to her breakfast and daily medicines is a nurse whom I learn comes regularly to help with the various activities of daily living, such as dressing, laundry, meals, and bathing. She also provides preventive and routine health care. These nursing services are administered by the city of Uppsala, Sweden's fourth-largest. Local governments are the principal providers for the nation's elderly. In-home care that allows Grandma to age in place is universally available in Sweden, a major factor in the nation's rank as the third-best country in the world in which to grow old according the Global AgeWatch Index.

The Global Age Watch employs four criteria to rank the well-being of those over sixty years of age in ninety-six countries: 1) *health outcomes*, including total life expectancy and healthy life expectancy at age sixty; 2) *income security*, including pension coverage, the old-age poverty rate, and measures of income and consumption of elderly people relative to the rest of the population; 3) *capability*, including the employment rate and educational attainment of elderly people; and 4) *enabling environment*, including measures of social integration, physical safety, civic freedom, and access to transportation. The United States ranks ninth in the Global AgeWatch Index, a far better performance than we have seen in previous chapters on comparative indices for infant, child, and working-age adult health outcomes.[1] This relatively strong US performance reflects a higher state commitment to the health of the elderly, namely through Social Security and Medicare. Medicaid, the US health coverage for low-income families, also plays a major role. In fact, one-fifth of Medicare's forty-four million beneficiaries, a number that is growing by ten thousand per day, also qualify for Medicaid assistance. Medicaid pays the fees for 63 percent of all nursing home residents, 54 percent of adult day service centers, 15 percent of those who live in residential care communities, and 9 percent of all home health agency fees. Although Medicaid was not originally created for such a role, it has become an essential component of America's system for providing health care to elderly people.

Despite the substantial combined efforts of Medicare, Medicaid, Social Security, and local and private programs, America's elderly suffer from health deficits that accumulate during childhood and their working years due to harmful social determinants, gaps in health care coverage, lack of attention to prevention, and lifestyle choices. As a result, America's elderly are sicker when compared to their counterparts in similar-income European nations. Population aging is among the most compelling challenges that the US health system faces, and it is aggravated by the poor social determinants that cumulatively affect Americans' health during their younger years.

The elderly of comparable-income European nations owe much of their stronger health outcomes to the positive influences, policies, and programs that have benefited them over their life course. To be sure, the institutions aimed specifically at the protection and promotion of elderly health are important, but they must be viewed in the context of life-course effects. For example, in the preceding chapter, we examined the historical evolution of Germany's efforts to promote and sustain the health of its working-age population. Those efforts pay off when Germans age into retirement. A 2017 Commonwealth Fund study examined the challenges faced by people sixty-five and older in eleven high-income countries. It found that 24 percent of elderly Germans suffer from three or more chronic diseases—the highest rate of any of the European nations examined. Yet Germany's rate is still only two-thirds the US rate. Fully 36 percent of US elderly people suffer from three or more chronic diseases, by far the largest share of the eleven countries examined. The United States looks even worse when compared to Sweden, especially when critical social determinants of health are included. Twenty-five percent of older Americans reported worrying about paying for housing, nutritious meals, utilities, and medical needs compared to only 4 percent of elderly Swedes. Fifteen percent of US elderly persons compared to 8 percent of elderly Swedes reported an emergency room visit that could have been avoided if timely and appropriate primary care services had been available. Only two percent of Sweden's elderly reported skipping care because of cost concerns versus 31 percent of older Americans.[2]

Though Medicare provides health coverage to over 90 percent of Americans aged sixty-five and older, additional insurance premiums, co-payments, and out-of-pocket expenses for physician services, prescription drugs, hearing devices, and dentistry continue to pose significant barriers to strong health outcomes. In contrast, Sweden caps cost-sharing for elderly patients at $120 per year. With no such cap, older Americans face both higher prices for medical services and prescription drugs—double or triple in many cases—than other high-income nations.[3] And the higher costs are not limited to individuals. Insufficient investment in social services and a failure to rectify negative social determinants such as insecure housing and barriers to mobility and nutritious food results in higher social costs, which are ultimately borne by the elderly and the Medicare and Medicaid programs. Such burdens could be alleviated if appropriate health coverage, prevention, and greater attention to the social determinants of health occurred earlier in the life course.[4]

Obesity, a serious medical condition that often develops early in the life course, is perhaps the most poignant example of the US health system's failure. Fully 42 percent of Americans between the ages of forty and fifty-nine, and 41 percent of those over fifty-nine are obese.[5] In contrast, Swedish public health leaders are alarmed because the obesity rate in their population between the ages of forty-five and eighty-five has ticked up in recent years to 19 percent, less than half the US rate.[6] And they have every right to be concerned. Research consistently links obesity with heightened risks of cardiovascular disease (heart failure, myocardial infarction, and stroke), diabetes, metabolic disorders, several cancers (especially of the colon, breast, and prostate), the exacerbation of osteoarthritis, rheumatoid arthritis, and gout, functional limitations, and disability. In the United States, virtually all of these obesity-linked health risks in the elderly are shouldered by federal and state programs, namely Medicare and Medicaid, even though their origins lie much earlier in the life course, when corrective actions could have avoided costly medical care and untold suffering in people's later years.

Before we proceed with our comparative historical inquiry into the social determinants of elderly health in Sweden and the United States, we must first examine what we mean by "elderly" and "old age." These terms are both historically contingent and socially constructed. For example, Great Britain's Friendly Societies Act of 1875, which regulated private pension annuities, defined old age as "any age" after fifty. Not ten year later, Chancellor Otto von Bismarck initially chose seventy as the age at which workers could receive a retirement pension under Germany's 1883 old-age insurance law; he eventually lowered the age of eligibility to sixty-five. In neither the British nor German case is there evidence that medical experts advised their respective governments when they selected these demarcations between "not old" and "old." Actuarial calculations dictated Bismarck's initial choice of seventy and political pressure led to its downward revision. Germany's choice of sixty-five has since become the most common normal retirement age across industrialized nations, including Sweden and the United States, although many offer reduced pensions earlier (at age sixty-one in Sweden and sixty-two in the United States). Several countries, including the United States, will raise their *normal retirement age*—a term that denotes eligibility for "full" pension benefits—by two or three years in the coming decade. Meanwhile, Japanese researchers, who have considered evidence from long-term longitudinal epidemiological, clinical, and pathological studies, recommend that the definition of *elderly* and eligibility for retirement benefits should be raised to age seventy-five. On the other hand, one might ask why eligibility for a retirement pension should determine who is considered old. The US Age Discrimination in Employment Act defines "older persons" as anyone over thirty-nine. Yet surveys reveal that most seventy-five-year-olds do not think they belong in the "old age" category.[7] And they may be right. Abundant research indicates that calendar age is not equivalent to biological age, especially when disaggregating populations by race, ethnicity, socioeconomic class, and gender. Finally, the notion of retirement itself is a social construction that only emerged with the advent of the industrial revolution, and it took several decades for it to become common. For the purposes of this chapter, despite the bluntness with which it captures the meaning of "elderly" and "old age," we will conform to the Bismarckian paradigm that continues to dominate aging policy (and data-gathering) in the United States and Europe. Though many persons well beyond the age of sixty-five remain active in the labor force, and many others cease work well before that age, our analysis will focus on those who have surpassed the age of sixty-four. Throughout, sex and gender will take center stage due to the feminization of old age on both sides of the Atlantic. Indeed, only seventy-seven men live beyond age sixty-five for every one hundred women in the United States, while eighty-one Swedish men survive past sixty-five for every hundred women in Sweden.[8] While women may experience longer lives, they are more likely to experience relatively poor income security, unstable housing, and other harmful social determinants of health, especially in the United States.

This chapter provides a historical comparison of public and private institutions and policies—local, regional, and national—that seek to ensure the health of the elderly in the United States and Sweden. I also pay particular attention to health care services, with an eye toward their influence both during old age and earlier in the life course. The World Health Organization has identified three broad social determinants as critical to healthy aging, and these serve to organize the chapter: 1) financial security, including the ability of the elderly to afford appropriate and safe housing, maintain a nutritious diet, and benefit from adequate means of transport; 2) social integration, the degree to which the elderly participate in the community, through continued employment, volunteering, or activity in clubs, sports, or other social organizations; and 3) access to preventive and curative health services, including long-term care, and the proximity of these services to the community in which the elderly live.[9] Most elderly persons in the United States and Sweden do not participate in the labor force and therefore rely more heavily on private savings, pensions, family members, and public provisions to preserve their well-being and health. In short, many are, by choice or not, retired. That being the case, any history of the social influences on elderly health must begin with a discussion of retirement itself: why and how it developed during the nineteenth and twentieth centuries and what role it plays in aging and health today.

Industrialism and the Creation of Retirement

The new production processes that began in Britain during the latter half of the eighteenth century—what historians call the Industrial Revolution—transformed the nature of work and thereby how we think about aging. The bulk of society's productive capacity moved away from human and animal muscles to machines, and from the countryside to the city. Powerful fossil-fuel energy replaced water wheels. New chemicals, advancements in steel production, electric motors, and the internal combustion engine made possible vast increases in productivity and a much greater variety of goods.[10] The scale of manufacturing facilities grew to previously unimagined size. In 1750, a factory that employed fifty workers would have been considered large. By 1900 the same factory would have been considered a mere workshop. Industrial plants now employed thousands, working in shifts around the clock. Industrialization also transformed our conception of speed and time itself. Distances shrank, first because of the railroad and the telegraph but also due to the bicycle and then the automobile—themselves products of the industrial age. Synchronized clocks proliferated as markets grew; once strictly local merchants now bought and sold their goods across nations, continents, and oceans. Like their compatriots, the elderly were no doubt awed by the availability of new products and the sheer speed of change. Yet, unlike their younger neighbors, many older people soon learned that they could not keep up with the accelerated pace of work inherent in industrial production.[11]

The new methods of mass production played to the strengths of youth. Rapid and tireless machines were most efficient when matched with speedy, dexterous, high-endurance workers. Social relations in the workplace also shifted. Unlike the workshops and farms of the pre-industrial era, relations between owner and employee became distant, even anonymous. Industrialists now sought to retire their older, less productive workers in much the same way they retired worn equipment. The fledgling workers' unions fought back, not against the forced unemployment of older workers, per se, but rather for a more humane manner of doing it.[12]

Thus was born the ternary life course to which the citizens of industrialized nations have grown accustomed: childhood, work, and retirement. Although retirement was invented in manufacturing, it spread to most sectors of the economy by the mid-twentieth century. Retirement is therefore a social construction of the first order, born of the wrenching changes to work wrought by the industrial revolution. Remarkably, retirement, whether forced or voluntary, became a cultural norm in less than two generations. As a result, social practices in housing, labor markets, and mass-market products evolved to service those who had entered what sociologists call the *third age*, usually beginning at age sixty-five, emphasizing its distinctiveness from the two earlier phases of the life course: childhood and work.[13] How the United States and Sweden each reacted to the plight of their older workers, especially those who first faced the specter of industrialization, provides an early indication of the value that each nation would attach to ensuring elderly health in succeeding generations.

Old-Age Financial Security: United States, 1890–1950

A machinist named James O'Connell learned the brutal nature of nineteenth-century industrialization as only a shop-floor worker could. Starting as an apprentice in his teens, he spent nearly forty years in manufacturing, rising to become president of the International Association of Machinists. Near the end of his life in 1906, O'Connell recalled the desperation of his fellow aging workers who experienced the industrial transformation of work firsthand. In sometimes emotional language, he described the quandary of an older expert machinist whose skill, regardless of his age, had previously "won him the respect of his shop mates, while this same skill, adding to the company profits, brought appreciation from his employers." All was well, O'Connell reflected, until "the speeding up of the machine." Unable to keep pace, the mature expert was "no longer profitable." And after "dismissal from one job, it [was] difficult, if not impossible, to get a job elsewhere." O'Connell bemoaned the commonness with which forty-year-old men, even those with apparently secure jobs, turned to hair dye to hide their age.[14] O'Connell's description of what machinists faced applied in spades to the less-skilled workers who, upon entering late middle age, struggled to keep pace with work on the factory floor. Some employers accommodated their older workers by shifting them to less demanding roles, such as work as night watchmen or custodians, although not without substantial pay cuts. But there were only so many of these less production-intensive posts to be had. Those who could retire did so, usually relying on family support and meager savings. Many nineteenth-century US manufacturing centers saw a sharp rise in the elderly among their neediest poverty-stricken residents, most of whom possessed no way to sustain themselves.[15] To the frustration of city leaders, the elderly poor were filling the almshouses and burdening municipal budgets.

The railroads, manufacturing, mining, and large commercial enterprises were the first to respond with pension plans as a solution to the falling productivity of older workers.[16] Pension plans first appeared in the 1880s, and by 1930 there were 370 plans across the United States, covering 15 percent of the private-sector labor force.[17] Eighty-seven percent of the largest two hundred US firms had pension plans of some kind by 1930. But only 2 percent of companies of less than 250 employees offered pensions, and most Americans worked for these companies or for themselves.[18] Industrial employers created pension plans for three principal reasons: to slow labor-force turnover, to facilitate the firing of less productive older workers, and to combat strikes. In order to gain benefits, an employee had to remain with the firm without interruption for between twenty and thirty years, which became known as the vesting period. This rule dissuaded high-skilled workers from switching firms in search of better pay. Upon reaching a specified advanced age, usually sixty-five, the employee faced mandatory retirement and was granted an annual pension, generally 1 percent of his or her average salary times the number of years in the company's service. The legal nature of the pension also meant that employers could use it to control both those still working and retirees.

Company retirement funds accepted no worker or union contributions and were solely administered by the employer. Thus, in the eyes of the courts, a pension constituted a gift from the employer to the employee, and, as such, the employer could revoke it at will. The following provision in Western Electric's pension plan was typical and served to discourage workers' participation in strikes or unauthorized work slowdowns: "No employee shall have a right . . . to any pension allowance and the company reserves its right and privilege to discharge any officer, agent or employee, when the interests of the company in its judgement may so require without any liability or any claim for a pension."[19] In fact, some pension plans permitted the company to recall pensioners to work, including to help break strikes. If a pensioner failed to respond to the recall, the firm could revoke his or her pension. Other firms used their pension plans to control employee behavior beyond the workplace. The First National Bank of Chicago expressly threatened to withdraw the pension and dismiss any "clerk who marries on a salary of less than $1,000 a year." A male employee convicted "for felony or misdemeanor" would lose his pension, while a widowed female employee could lose hers even in the absence of a conviction if the misconduct were "proved to the satisfaction of the bank."[20]

As described in the preceding chapter, German chancellor Otto von Bismarck created old-age social insurance in 1883 in an attempt to sever the bond between Germany's Social Democratic Party and the country's industrial workers. In the United States, there existed no comparably powerful socialist party, which might have militated for state action to protect workers from imperious employers. Beginning in the 1890s, unions created their own pension plans, financed by member dues. These efforts were most common in the skilled-craft unions, such as the building trades, electrical work, and printing—all of which, like most craft unions, excluded African Americans, immigrants, and women. By 1930, union plans covered some 20 percent of their members, but few were able to achieve the levels of income-replacement benefits offered by the company plans. One of the most powerful union leaders, Samuel Gompers of the American Federation of Labor, actively opposed German-style old-age pensions or any government initiative that would impinge on the union's autonomy. Without widespread adherence or government support, union pension plans often resembled fraternal society benefits, providing only life and disability insurance and payments to widows. These were undoubtedly lifesaving benefits for some, but they did not provide for the well-being in old age that many European workers were winning.[21] As private pensions and mandatory retirement spread across the US industrial and commercial sectors, state and federal governments adopted their own plans.[22]

In 1918, Lewis Meriam of the Institute for Government Research—the precursor of today's Brookings Institution—wrote an influential report that advocated a different approach for the public sector. Meriam clearly appreciated the strengths of European old-age social insurance though he insisted that a single retirement age for all employees would be inappropriate given their differing kinds of work. "Unfortunately," Meriam wrote, "an ideal retirement age for policemen and firemen, for example, would be anything but ideal if applied to clerks." But he also noted that the government ought to eschew the bald labor-control devices that were prevalent in private company plans. Private employers' motives for creating pension plans stemmed from company interests, but Meriam concluded that a retirement system should systematically provide "for the care of the old and disabled eliminated from the public service and possibly to a limited extent for the care of the dependents of deceased public employees."[23] Here we see the early divergence between private- and public-sector approaches to the provision of financial security for the elderly.

On one side stood industrial and commercial employers whose pension plans were motivated by labor-force control, productivity, and company profits. On the other side stood a civil service model that was adopted by many states and cities. It recognized the larger social implications of retirement policy. Both models advocated pensions for older workers in order to maintain productivity, but the civil service model showed broader concern for the elderly workers' financial security. The civil service model also recognized superannuated workers as family breadwinners. In the view of proponents, any mandatory retirement system ought to keep not just retirees but also dependent family members, especially wives, out of the almshouses, a social determinant of health for which most private plans appeared to care little.

Indeed, elderly women bore the brunt of suffering in the newly industrialized economy of the early twentieth century. A relatively low male life expectancy, the widespread practice of paying women less (even for identical work), and low divorce rates meant that women who survived past midlife commonly lived out their lives in financial precarity. In 1910,

20 percent of ever-married women over age fifty were widows; the proportion rose to 50 percent for those aged sixty-five to sixty-nine. Some 30 percent of these remained active in the labor force until they reached seventy. But after age seventy less than 10 percent could continue to work, no matter their level of familial support. In order to afford housing, 72 percent of widows lived with others, often an adult child or a fellow tenant with whom they could share expenses to stretch their meager savings. Approximately one-quarter of widows ended up in public boardinghouses with few amenities and little care. If elderly men, unable to keep pace with factory machines, were cast off like obsolete tools, their surviving spouses suffered as much or more. They either fell into the dependency of their children or were forced into boardinghouses that were ill equipped to care for them. From these boardinghouses grew the nursing homes of today's US eldercare system. And, true to their origins, the ability of these new institutions to offer quality care to their still mostly female residents varies widely. Indeed, already by the mid-twentieth century, the health outcomes of elderly Americans, a large majority of whom were women, were falling behind their European counterparts.[24]

Yet, in 1920, Americans who advocated German-style old-age social insurance risked being labeled a German sympathizer or a communist. With the First World War still in recent memory and the communist revolution in Russia underway, few braved such un-American labels.[25] Besides, technological innovation, nearly full employment, and vibrant economic growth seemed to have vindicated the values of individual liberty and self-help, at least for the young. Indeed, mortality rates for US working-age adults fell between 1900 and 1920.[26] Private and civil service pension plans continued to gain adherents, and the most powerful labor unions remained committed to building their own pension programs. Moreover, the commercial insurers who sold life and disability insurance opposed government intervention that would disrupt their business. By the late 1920s, some 2,700,000 public- and private-sector workers—10 percent of the labor force—were covered by some sort of pension, and the number was rising at ever-greater annual rates. This allowed the proponents of voluntarism to prevent any serious consideration of state-led measures that were being enacted in Europe.[27] As long as one ignored the brutal segregation of African Americans and discrimination against immigrants, the term "roaring" aptly captured the spirit of the 1920s. White women could now vote, and, much to the chagrin of social conservatives, many insisted on bicycling and driving automobiles, both of which were becoming common on US streets. Anything appeared possible in the exuberance of the 1920s—cars, airplanes, art deco skyscrapers—if only government would stay out of the way. When the crash came in 1929, it was first considered irrational and surely to be short-lived. Yet by 1932 the rhetoric of individual steadfastness to fight the Great Depression, promising that prosperity was just around the corner—President Herbert Hoover's favorite refrain, rang false in the face of a persistent national catastrophe.

In a remarkable about-face in US economic and social policy, newly elected president Franklin Roosevelt announced forceful state action to combat an unprecedented 25.2 percent unemployment rate in 1932. His New Deal would pick up where individual savings and voluntary organizations had failed. For the working-age unemployed, Roosevelt created jobs programs, such as the Works Progress Administration and the Civilian Conservation Corps. For the elderly, the New Deal meant passage of the 1935 Social Security Act, a pension program intended to vacate some elderly from the labor force, thereby making room for younger workers while ensuring a modicum of financial security for the elderly.

In 1934, Roosevelt established the Committee on Economic Security, which he charged with preparing a program for "National Social and Economic Security." The term "security," especially covering financial security in old age, had long been on the agenda of US reformers, including Roosevelt's incoming secretary of labor, Frances Perkins, who came from New York to the White House with Roosevelt. Populist movements that advocated old-age pensions were growing in strength across the country. Notably, a California physician and public health officer named Francis Townsend promised to end the Depression by paying stipends to older people. He boasted two million followers, a fifth of all those over sixty, who had enrolled in local "Townsend chapters" across the nation. Townsend called for a monthly payment of $200 to all those over age fifty-nine. In return, recipients had to retire and spend their stipends within one month, thereby spiking consumer demand, which would lead to the reopening of factories and businesses.[28] Roosevelt viewed Townsend and others like him as impracticable and instructed his Committee on Economic Security to draft legislation that closely resembled existing European social insurance and poverty relief.

Indeed, the Social Security Act of 1935 created a public pension plan that resembled German old-age insurance. Social Security's old-age benefits program funded pensions, starting at age sixty-five, and relied on a 2 percent payroll tax, split evenly between the employer and the employee, on the first $3,000 of earned income. (The Social Security payroll tax is still evenly shared by workers and employers and now stands at 12.4 percent on the first $127,200 dollars in earned income.)[29] This flat-rate payroll tax is regressive because it takes a greater share of low-wage workers' disposable income than that of high-income earners during their working years. However, a progressive calculation of benefits restores some of that share during retirement. For example, in 2018, a worker who earned only 45 percent of the average wage throughout her career would receive a pension with a value of 50 percent of prior earnings. Whereas, a high earner, whose gross pay amounted to 160 percent of the average wage during her working years, would receive pension benefits of 55 percent of prior earnings.[30] Initially, neither spouses nor dependents could collect benefits of a diseased beneficiary, but they were added to the law in 1939. Given the imperative of reducing poverty in the teeth of the Great Depression, the Social Security Act also included the Old Age Assistance program, which provided additional means-tested help to the very poor in partnership with the states on a fifty-fifty matching basis. The Social Security Act further included a modest unemployment insurance plan that was likewise funded by employer and worker payroll taxes.[31]

What is most striking about the 1935 Social Security Act is its exclusion of approximately half of the labor force. It left out agricultural workers, domestic service workers, the self-employed, and employees of religious, charitable, and educational organizations. As we saw in the previous chapter, racial discrimination explains the exclusion of farm and domestic service workers. In fact, those two exclusions alone made ineligible fully 90 percent of working-age African Americans who lived in the southern states and half of all black workers nationwide. Roosevelt's coalition of conservative Democrats from the South and Southwest simultaneously prevented the law's drafters from including health coverage in the Social Security Act because it would have required equal access to health care for whites and blacks.[32]

The Social Security Act also discriminated against women through its exclusion of charitable and educational workers. In a sharply gendered labor market where the high-paying jobs in commerce and industry were reserved for men, women disproportionately comprised the personnel of hospitals and schools. But with the law's exclusion of religious, charitable, and educational institutions, many nurses and teachers were banned from participation in Social Security. In old age they were instead shunted toward state poverty relief and the Old Age Assistance program, both of which were means-tested, with strict income thresholds. Women also suffered from the law's promotion of private labor markets. Social Security benefits were calculated so as to avoid the disruption of wage levels. No matter how long one contributed at any level, benefits rarely competed with the wage income from remaining employed. And uncompensated household labor, such as childcare, cooking, and housecleaning, which commonly fell to women, counted for nothing toward Social Security's old-age benefits. In this way, the new law reinforced the traditional male-breadwinner model, which left women, who commonly outlived their husbands, dependent on their husbands' contributions. For women who remained independent but were unable to break into more highly compensated, male-dominated job sectors, the 1935 Social Security Act brought virtually no improvement to their financial security in old age.[33] Ultimately, Social Security pensions constituted a poor replica of German old-age insurance because it excluded vast numbers of American workers along racial, ethnic, and gendered lines. Meanwhile, its relatively low benefits prevented it from replacing private-sector pensions. Private retirement plans remained active in many sectors of the US economy and, as we will see, would rekindle in ways even more threatening to the health of the elderly later in the century.

Old-Age Financial Security: Sweden, 1870–1950

Prior to the mid-nineteenth century, Sweden was among the poorest countries in Europe, its per capita GDP only 40 percent of Great Britain's. However, between 1890 and 1970 the Swedish economy grew seventeenfold, an achievement matched only by Japan in the modern era. By 1970, Sweden had become the fourth richest nation in the world behind Switzerland, the United States, and Luxembourg. Much of this fantastic growth was fueled by the sale of iron ore and timber to industrializing nations, notably Great Britain and Germany, that were hungry for natural resources. Many resource-rich countries fall prey to what economists call the "resource curse," whereby possession of rich natural endowments provokes conflict among rival elites and the spread of corruption, which obstructs economic growth and development. But solid legislation and institutions, including agricultural land reform, secure property rights, press freedoms, and equal inheritance rights for women and men, helped Sweden avoid the resource curse. The country remained neutral in both world wars, avoiding a German invasion in the second by agreeing to export iron ore to the Nazi Reich. So, like the United States after 1945, the nation's mines, factories, shipbuilding yards, and transport and commercial infrastructure stood unharmed by aerial bombardment. Swedish industries quickly expanded to meet the demand from war-torn nations in Europe and Asia to rebuild in the 1950s and 1960s.[34] Yet Sweden's efforts to ensure the health of its elderly began well before its post–World War II prosperity. Indeed, they began in the depths of poverty and despair.

Between 1870 and 1900, fully 16 percent of Sweden's 4,200,000 people emigrated to the United States. The emigrants were disproportionately young and the nation's most productive workers. Their departure made Sweden into the oldest country in the world in less than a generation. As a proportion of the national population, Sweden in 1900 had twice as many people over age sixty-five than England, Russia, Germany, or Austria. Families, churches, and local governments struggled to cope with the growing numbers of dependent elderly. National poverty laws compelled local authorities to provide relief to their elderly residents, but in order to do so they had to raise taxes on an ever-shrinking number of working-age adults. Churches emerged as the locus of poor relief and lodging, but their efforts remained insufficient and unsustainable under the strain of emigration.

Into this context came news of Germany's creation of social insurance in the 1880s, which sparked considerable interest and debate in Sweden. Adolf Hedin, a member of the Swedish Parliament, enthusiastically endorsed German-style social insurance and crafted legislation to emulate it. But his opponents accurately pointed out that Sweden was at a much earlier stage of industrialization than Germany. They argued that Sweden could ill afford the employer and worker payroll taxes that would fund social insurance. Now was not the moment, they said, to tax entrepreneurship, which would be critical to the expansion of Sweden's fledgling industries. Moreover, opponents insisted, why should industrial workers gain social benefits when (still in the 1880s) a much larger portion of Sweden's labor force than Germany's worked on farms. Faced with the power of rural representatives in the Riksdag—the Swedish Parliament—Hedin conceded that rural workers and farmers had to be included in any social reforms. In these debates we have the first indication that Sweden would create a new kind of welfare state, the *folkhemmet* ("people's home"), which would ultimately prove every bit as successful as German-style social insurance in improving the social determinants of health and spurring economic growth.[35]

Swedish lawmakers who supported a social safety net believed that Bismarck had it backwards. He had begun with health coverage in 1883, followed by accident insurance in 1884, waiting until 1889 to institute meager old-age pensions. Because destitute elderly lay at the center of Sweden's crisis, reformers enacted old-age pensions first, followed by health and accident insurance in due time. Moreover, because the problem of elder poverty spanned rural and urban regions, reformers from the Agrarian and Social Democratic Parties tapped the nation's progressive income tax, which had been created in 1902, to finance the new old-age pensions.[36]

Local municipalities remained central to the provision of benefits, but the pension law of 1913 demonstrated the financial efficiency of an income tax to assure intergenerational social support. Swedes funded the entirety of the new pension system by paying an additional earmarked portion on their income taxes. Eligibility began at age sixty-seven, although the advent of disability permitted access at a younger age. Because the additional pension tax sat atop an already progressive income tax, individuals likewise contributed to their pension along progressive lines; those with higher incomes paid substantially more but also earned a higher pension in retirement. Even then, this world's first universal pension system produced only enough revenue to rescue local governments from insolvency and keep the elderly out of the almshouses. It could not provide the same kind of financial security that employed working-age citizens enjoyed.[37] Nevertheless, enactment of universal pensions opened the way for the funding of other social safety net programs.[38] It also demonstrated the promise of a rural-urban political alliance.

Rural and urban political leaders had come together to rescue local municipalities from the burden of elder poverty. This alliance continued to shape the health policies of Sweden for decades to come. The Social Democratic Party grew its membership by reaching out to rural residents even as its working-class base grew apace with the nation's cities. The Social Democrats of the 1920s construed *folkhemmet* to mean that the nation had to provide for the health and security of all its members. This differed from the initial impetus of German social insurance, which was concerned first and foremost with the urban industrial working class; only later was it extended to the commercial and agricultural sectors. Also, Sweden's use of the income tax (rather than payroll taxes) permitted a relatively rapid universalization of benefits. This made irrelevant the fact that the nation's elderly, who had never paid into the system, were the first and greatest beneficiaries of the new pension. The "people's home" approach enabled Sweden to avoid the nettlesome issue of who was "deserving" and who was "less deserving" of benefits. As historian Sven Hort notes, the democratic roots of Sweden's welfare state made it "simultaneously less despotic, less étatist, and less elitist" than in Germany, where the throne, acting through Bismarck, had created social insurance primarily as a tool to undercut support for a growing socialist movement.[39]

In contrast to the top-down birth of Germany's welfare state, the urban and rural political accord that made possible an income-tax-funded old-age pension appears decidedly populist. From 1932 through the Second World War and beyond, Social Democrats and the Agrarian Party joined in a "Red-Green alliance." They collaborated to create a thick social safety net beyond pensions, with many child and family programs, including maternity benefits, childbirth services, housing subsidies for families with children, and generous government loans to newly married couples. Yet the commitment to ensure the financial security of the elderly never wavered. Most telling is the central place that pension reforms continued to occupy in Swedish politics, first in 1946 and then again in 1960 when deadlocked parliamentary leaders called a national referendum solely to settle a pension question they could not settle themselves. Indeed, the innovative reforms of the postwar years indicate that elderly health remained, as historian Hort puts it, "the core provision" of the country's welfare state.[40]

Because the 1913 pension law had been built atop a progressive income tax, higher income earners contributed more and enjoyed much higher pensions. The debate over reform centered on how best to alleviate the growing disparity between high-income and low-income elderly. Swedes rejected the creation of an American-style means-tested benefit to raise the pensions of low-income beneficiaries, which would have mirrored US Social Security Old Age Assistance. Instead, in order to avoid what economist Johannes Hagen calls "the demoralizing consequences of mean-tested benefits," they chose a universal flat-rate annual supplement of one thousand *krona* and a cash housing subsidy for elderly who lived in expensive regions, both funded by an additional 1 percent charge on income.[41] Yet by the late 1950s it once again became clear that even though the pension reform had eliminated old-age poverty, inequality among the elderly continued to grow. This forced a second round of reform in 1960.[42] In that year, a razor-thin referendum result permitted the Social Democrats to enact a supplemental earnings-related pension, known as the ATP (Allmänna Tilläggspensionen), that was paid to current workers. Within a few years, the ATP, operating alongside the flat-rate *folkpension*, found widespread support. Yet, as we will see, the ATP's reliance on a large and steady flow of contributions from current workers made it unsustainable when the Swedish economy slowed in the 1980s.[43]

Health and Long-Term Care, 1950–Present

Sweden possesses a unitary national government that delegates substantial power over health and welfare to regional and local authorities. The nation's twelve county councils have long administered all of the nation's hospitals, having been granted their ownership by the national government in 1862. The county councils and their associated municipalities, therefore, constitute the most important sources of health care services.

After the Second World War, the Swedish health care system underwent dramatic changes that helped the nation achieve some of the best population health outcomes in the world by the 1980s. In 1950, only half of Swedes had health coverage, primarily through mutual benefit societies. Their means-tested premiums focused on the replacement of lost wages and offered only modest reimbursement for doctors' fees and pharmaceuticals. As the effectiveness of medical care increased in the mid-twentieth century, the price of in-patient and ambulatory care quickly outstripped the mutual benefit societies' ability to cover medical expenses. In 1955, a Social Democratic–led government created universal public health coverage. Like the 1913 pension program, income tax revenues paid for the newly enacted universal health care plan. By 1968, the plan covered 80 percent of the health care expenses of all Swedes.

The rapid growth in importance of publicly funded health coverage led to a showdown with the nation's physicians who remained in private practice, billing on a fee-for-service basis. In most cases they were also employed by county hospitals and operated their private practices within them. Thus, patients paid their doctors directly and then sought reimbursement from the public health plan. Yet the system became unwieldy as the price of health services rose. Studies indicated that therapies were warped toward in-patient care, largely because 80 percent of doctors worked in county hospitals. In response, in 1970 the national government passed the "seven-crown reform," so-called because seven *krona* ($1.35 in 1970) became the standard copayment for out-patient services. But the reform went well beyond copayments.

The county councils and municipalities assumed full administrative control of out-patient services. Many physicians abandoned their private practices to accept salaried positions in the hospitals; others established private ambulatory-care clinics or offices outside the hospitals and then negotiated fee schedules with the county governments. In the following year, 1971, the national government similarly brought the nation's pharmacies under pubic control and some years later handed responsibility for them to the county councils. In 1974, the nation's public health coverage added dental care to its services. With a full spectrum of ambulatory and in-patient care assets under their control and universal coverage in place, county governments systematically coordinated the nation's public health and social services, pharmaceutical delivery, dental care, and primary and specialty medical treatment. This coordination of health services included home and long-term care for the nation's elderly.[44] At about this same time the United States faced a crisis in elderly health as the growth of private health insurance coverage stalled.

In 1960, observers across the political spectrum agreed that the US health system had hit what might be called a 75 percent plateau. Employer-provided coverage accounted for 75 percent of all health insurance enrollees. Employers and their workers paid 75 percent of all health insurance premiums. And the Health Insurance Institute—an industry trade organization—estimated that 136,000,000 Americans, or about 75 percent of the population, possessed some form of health insurance.[45] Much of the unionized working class and most middle- and upper-class professionals—along with their dependents—enjoyed health coverage. Yet here the spread of private health insurance had stalled. Large swaths of the elderly, having left the labor force, now lacked the all-important link with employment on which US health coverage had been built. Many low- and middle-income elderly appeared destined to remain forever outside the private health insurance system. In 1962, President John Kennedy oversaw the development of plans to solve the problem. In 1965, a fully developed proposal to create national public health insurance for the US elderly, Medicare, entered the political fray.

Better than anyone, private health insurers understood the technical reason why the nation's elderly needed public health insurance: experience-rated policy writing had taken over the health insurance industry. The price of insurance, whether for an employer group or for an individual, had become closely linked to the medical histories and health care use records of the beneficiaries. The elderly exhibited high morbidity and high rates of health care use, which drove up their premiums. Only the exceptional private employer or union could afford to include retirees, and many elderly had access to neither.[46] Indeed, large airlines and major employers in steelmaking and automobile manufacture were trimming retiree benefits, not adding to them.[47] Like in Sweden, health care costs were on the rise because of new and effective but expensive medical therapies and technologies. Hospitals were on the front lines of medical care for the elderly; they were seeing a marked rise in uncompensated care because more and more elderly patients lacked insurance. As one American Hospital Association administrator put it, "An increasing number of hospitals became ready to accept the Social Security [Medicare] principle because they could see no other way to get the needed money."[48] Employers and union leaders alike had also come around to the idea that public health insurance for the elderly was the best solution. In fact, a White House phone recording indicates that Lyndon Johnson personally persuaded AFL-CIO president George Meany to join the Medicare cause.[49] All of these stakeholders—insurers, hospitals, employers, and unions—feared a large-scale government intervention in the health care system that would upend the generous benefits and handsome profits that the private health insurance system provided. However, US physicians stood outside this growing consensus. Unlike their Swedish counterparts, they fought hard to prevent the creation of public health coverage for the elderly. As we saw in chapter 1, they were also unwilling to negotiate a grand bargain with the government like French doctors had done in 1928, protecting private-practice medicine and patient choice.

Instead, American Medical Association president Leonard Larson warned that the enactment of Medicare would be the first step toward "socialized medicine," leading to "a disruption in the doctor-patient relationship, delays in admissions to hospitals; waiting lists for various operations and therapies; regimentation in medical practice . . . in other words, medicine in action on a government run, assembly line basis." Larson's view of Medicare relied on an AMA board member who had visited Great Britain to study the National Health Service (NHS). He concluded that it was "becoming more and more distasteful to the people—the patients and the physicians . . . [and] is still being plagued with rising costs, greater inconveniences, increasing governmental redtape, and a diminishing quality of medical care."[50] However, the AMA's focus on Great Britain was irrelevant. The NHS truly was (and is) a socialized system of health care delivery under which most providers work for the government; it had little in common with the Medicare proposal.

AMA leaders of the early 1960s clearly hoped to repeat the victory they had won over President Franklin Roosevelt's attempt to include health insurance in the 1935 Social Security Act, this time against President Lyndon Johnson. The AMA launched the largest and most expensive publicity campaign ever undertaken by a private organization in the United States. It sought to discredit the Medicare proposal as "socialized medicine" that would "destroy the concepts of individual and family responsibility." The AMA bought quarter-page ads in seven thousand dailies, full-page ads in every major metropolitan newspaper and most major weeklies, thirty one-minute spots on national television, and hundreds more local television ads. Ronald Reagan, then a B-list Hollywood actor, served as the AMA's principal spokesman in the TV ads.[51] But the political winds on health care had shifted dramatically since the 1930s when the AMA had prevailed over Roosevelt.

Private health coverage had grown into a tangle of powerful interests and beneficiaries, producing many winners. They included hospitals, insurers, salaried employees, and workers in union-organized sectors of the economy who enjoyed generous health care benefits. Above all, these winners wished to protect the system from radical reform; they believed that Medicare and the accompanying Medicaid proposal would do just that. Worse, the AMA leadership had seriously misjudged President Johnson. Formerly a long-time member of Congress, he understood that even a formidable adversary—and there were few more powerful lobbies than the AMA at the time—could be defeated if isolated. Drawing on his Texas farm-country upbringing, Johnson confided to AFL-CIO head George Meany to explain his view of the AMA's circumstances: "Have you ever fed chickens? . . . Chickens are real dumb. They eat and eat and eat and they never stop. Why they start shitting at the same time they're eating, and before you know it, they're knee-deep in their own shit. Well, the AMA's the same. They've been eating and eating nonstop and now they're knee-deep in their own shit and everybody knows it."[52] Johnson correctly surmised that the AMA's campaign against Medicare would fail if employers, unions, the hospitals, and the health insurers remained on the political sidelines. And he knew that Representative Wilbur Mills, Democrat from Louisiana and the chair of the powerful House Ways and Means Committee, had crafted a Medicare bill that could do just that.

Mills's bill, which one health official called a "three-layer cake," became an amendment to the 1935 Social Security Act. The top layer consisted of hospital insurance for the elderly (Medicare Part A), funded through a small increase in the Social Security payroll tax. Coverage for medical services (Medicare Part B) constituted the middle layer and was paid for by beneficiaries' premiums and the federal treasury. Medicaid, the federal-state program that provided means-tested health coverage for poor people, provided the bottom layer of the cake. Mill's Medicare bill gained overwhelming approval in both the House (307–116) and the Senate (70–24), and Johnson signed the measure into law in July 1965.[53] Within a few years, it became clear that the AMA's dire predictions about the nation's decline into socialism in the event that Medicare became law had been utterly wrong.

Indeed, Medicare embraced the liberties of fee-for-service medical practice. It adopted physicians' prevailing billing practices, known as "usual, customary, and reasonable," whose inflationary effects on health care costs are now well known. Likewise, Medicare reimbursed hospital services for the elderly on a "cost-plus" basis; hospitals simply calculated the price of their services and tacked on a significant percentage of the total to cover depreciation of plant and equipment. During the first year of Medicare's implementation alone, physician fees rose 7.8 percent, and hospital charges were up 16.5 percent—double the increases of previous years.[54] Not until the 1980s did Medicare put an end to the profligate spending of public money by unregulated medical providers. Ironically, when Medicare finally reined in costs of health care for the elderly through the creation of Diagnosis-Related Groups (DRG) payments to hospitals and value-based pricing for physician services, Ronald Reagan, once the AMA's chief spokesperson against Medicare, sat in the White House, directing the action.[55]

Prior to the creation of Medicare, only 46 percent of America's elderly possessed hospital insurance. Within a few years of its passage, 96 percent of those sixty-five or older had enrolled in Medicare Part A or Part B.[56] Despite this fantastic improvement in coverage, Medicare remains modest compared to the health care access afforded to Sweden's elderly. Few US elderly people fail to meet Medicare's eligibility threshold: ten years of employment, paying the Medicare payroll tax of 1.45 percent for those earning less than $250,000 per year. It is not eligibility but rather Medicare's substantial cost-sharing requirements that threaten the financial security of many US elderly.

Medicare coverage for medical services (Part B) requires a monthly $135 premium and leaves 20 percent of costs to the beneficiary, with no lifetime limit. In contrast to Sweden's universal and comprehensive health coverage, Medicare does not cover dental, vision, and hearing devices, and until 2003 it did not cover prescription drugs. Because half of all Medicare beneficiaries have annual incomes below $26,200, even a relatively simple outpatient surgery can pose a substantial strain to many beneficiaries' financial security and hence their overall health. Indeed, when all is accounted, Medicare beneficiaries who remain in what is now called the traditional program pay about half of their total health care costs from their own savings.[57] Private insurers have stepped in to fill this breach, creating entirely new health insurance sectors, but this has created problems of its own.

Private insurers sell supplemental insurance that covers beneficiaries' 20 percent copayment for physician services. Indeed, some 30 percent of traditional Medicare beneficiaries possessed one of these so-called

Medi-gap plans in 2016.[58] In contrast to their Swedish counterparts, Americans who rely on private supplemental plans face age discrimination. Insurers cannot legally raise rates because of a subscriber's use of medical services, but they may raise premiums as the beneficiary ages, so that, for example, a California Blue Shield Medicare supplemental plan for a woman over eighty-five cost approximately $4,800 per year in 2019.[59] Beneficiaries who cannot afford supplemental plans seek coverage under means-tested programs for the poor, namely Medicaid. However, depending on the state, Medicaid requires a beneficiary to "spend down": eligibility is obtained only after the elderly person has expended most of her savings and liquidated all assets except a home and an automobile (if they have one). For example, a Medicaid recipient in New York State cannot possess more than $15,450 in total savings, whether checking, stocks, bonds, or retirement accounts.[60] In other words, older people are compelled to impoverish themselves to gain access to adequate health coverage, thus further undermining their health (financial security is one of the most important social determinants of health).

A more recent development in private insurance for Medicare beneficiaries, one that has accelerated in recent years, is the creation of Medicare Advantage plans. Under Medicare Advantage, a private insurer collects the Medicare beneficiary's Part B premium. In exchange, the beneficiary gains access to a closed network of medical providers who are contracted with the insurer. Although the network restricts patient choice of provider, the Medicare Advantage plans are popular and now cover about 30 percent of all Medicare beneficiaries. Patients are not responsible for the 20 percent copayment for medical services required in the traditional Medicare program. Also, many Medicare Advantage plans offer coverage for dentistry, vision services, hearing aids, and prescription drugs at modest prices. Unfortunately, the Medicare Advantage plans have greatly exacerbated health care inequities, notably between urban and rural residents.

Because insurers are not required to create nationwide Medicare Advantage provider networks, they have only done so in the most profitable regions of the country, usually in and near urban centers. For example, in Dade County, Florida—Miami—two-thirds of Medicare beneficiaries are enrolled in Medicare Advantage plans, but in nearly 25 percent of all other US counties, which are overwhelmingly rural and relatively poor, 0–10 percent of Medicare beneficiaries select Advantage plans. That is because either no provider network exists there or the network is so thinly constructed that a beneficiary would have to travel long distances to obtain care.[61] All this considered, Medicare's high out-of-pocket costs and serious access limitations are not its worst shortcomings. Medicare's greatest inadequacy compared to Sweden's elderly health care system concerns long-term care.

Whether provided in the home or at a nursing facility, long-term care includes help with the activities of daily living (ADLs): eating, bathing, dressing, toileting, and grooming as well as simple health care (e.g., the administering of eye drops).[62] Although ADLs are similar across the two nations, the American and Swedish health systems diverge drastically in their support of long-term care. Medicare simply ignores its important influence on health and refuses to pay for it. It defines long-term care as non-medical and "custodial" unless it is directly necessary for treatment after an acute medical event, such as a cerebrovascular accident (stroke). Medicare further medicalizes its home-care coverage by requiring that the beneficiary be physically homebound and under a physician's treatment plan. Even then, Medicare-covered home-care services typically cannot exceed three weeks in duration and cannot include delivered meals or assistance with other imperatives of home living, such as shopping, cleaning, and laundry.[63] The 1965 Older Americans Act provides means-tested home-care subsidies to the neediest elderly, but its funding has been flat over the last decade, failing to keep pace with inflation and the rising demand from the rapidly expanding elderly population.[64] Higher-income elderly can afford to purchase private long-term care insurance, but all but the most expensive policies exclude reimbursement for the first ninety days of need and then only cover a maximum of three years of care. Therefore, most policies charge premiums well above average expected benefits and provide limited coverage relative to the total expenditure risk.[65]

In contrast, the Swedish health system views full-spectrum long-term care as an essential determinant of elderly people's health. It provides universal and comprehensive care coverage, irrespective of any direct association with a medical event. In other words, a large percentage of elderly Americans who need sustained assistance with the activities of daily living cannot rely on Medicare, the very health program that was expressly created for them in 1965. Instead, they must turn to Medicaid, which, as we have seen, requires low income and asset levels to qualify. Little wonder that Medicaid has become the primary payer for long-term care in the United States, covering 60 percent of all nursing home residents nationwide. While Medicaid covers some in-home services, 70 percent of its spending on long-term care goes to nursing homes.[66] In contrast, when Swedes talk about "home help," they are not just referring to assistance with the activities of daily living.

They are talking about Sweden's Home Help program, created in the 1970s, which provides 24/7 support to older persons who are aging at home. It is free to low-income elderly people and available for a modest fee to those of higher incomes. (The maximum payment in 2016 was $126 per year.) Home Help includes transportation services, personal alarm systems, home-delivered meals, and assistance with the activities of daily living. Elderly Swedes' greater levels of financial security in old age (afforded by the previously discussed national pension system) and their universal access to quality health care during their childhood and working-age years, combined with Home Help, contribute to very high levels of elderly health outcomes. Indeed, a cross-national comparison of the so-called "old-old" (those over seventy-four years of age), revealed that the proportion of Americans who need help with ADLs is twice as large as their Swedish counterparts; and a far greater proportion of Americans over seventy-four require assistance with multiple activities of daily living, rather than just one, as is the case in Sweden.[67] Better elderly health, including among the old-old, makes "aging in place" possible on a larger scale in Sweden than in the United States. For those who do not own or cannot afford to rent a home or apartment after retirement, Sweden's Home Help program also provides housing subsidies; research indicates that secure, safe housing is a foundational social determinant of health. Indeed, 30 percent of older Swedes receive housing subsidies in some form.[68]

Overall, Swedish municipalities invest considerable resources in elder care; some 24 percent of people sixty-five or older receive assistance so they may live at home. And the nation as a whole expends 3.6 percent of its GDP on eldercare. Sweden's integration of local social welfare services with primary, specialty, and long-term care helps to explain why Sweden demonstrates some of the best health outcomes and the lowest levels of unmet need among dependent older people in the world.[69]

Social Integration, 1960–Present

As noted previously, social integration is the degree to which the elderly participate in the community through continued employment, volunteering, or activity in clubs, sports, or other social organizations. Through these activities the elderly build what is known as "social capital." A growing research literature indicates that social capital constitutes a substantial positive influence on health outcomes, including lower levels of depression and functional impairment, and reduced risk of mortality. These findings are especially relevant to elderly persons who have left the labor force, where many people fulfill most of their daily social interactions.[70] Political scientist Robert Putman distinguishes between two kinds of activities that build an individual's social capital: "bonding" and "bridging." Bonding refers to close interpersonal relations, most often with family members and good friends who constitute one's "inner circle." Meanwhile, bridging refers to social relations that are nourished outside the inner circle among people who vary in sociodemographic traits, such as age, class, race, and ethnicity. Another important social capital researcher, Ichiro Kawichi, stresses an ecological dimension. Social capital, he says, "should be properly considered a feature of the collective (neighborhood, community, society) to which the individual belongs."[71] Indeed, most research indicates that bridging social activities, those outside of one's inner circle, have the greatest positive effects on health outcomes, including reduced mortality rates.[72]

Yet the ability of older people to initiate and maintain social activities outside their inner circle may itself be dependent on their health. For example, if an individual lacks adequate mobility or hearing, she may be unable to engage in bridging activities. Therefore, access to health care services, such as hearing aid provision and physical therapy, to ensure sufficient functional abilities constitutes an important social determinant of health. Moreover, if a substantial portion of an elderly community's members cannot obtain health services, the community may itself become collectively less capable of maintaining the social capital of its members. As we have seen, in contrast to Sweden's comprehensive health coverage and Home Help program, Medicare does not systematically cover transportation services or hearing aids. This creates health disparities for

American elderly who suffer from hearing loss or mobility limitations. Those of higher socioeconomic position can purchase the needed services out-of-pocket or afford a supplemental insurance plan that covers them. They join Medicare beneficiaries who happen to reside in urban areas where a comprehensive Medicare Advantage plan may include hearing devices. But, as we have seen, only about a third of Medicare beneficiaries are enrolled in Medicare Advantage plans, half have annual incomes less than $26,200; and 25 percent possess total savings—retirement accounts and other financial assets—below $15,000.[73] Further, the housing choices and facilities where the elderly live influence the potential for social integration.

First among these are the bridging opportunities provided by intergenerational and aging-friendly communities. In this regard, the Americans and Swedes face quite different challenges. Because Sweden's universal and comprehensive health system for the elderly makes possible aging in place, 90 percent of those over age sixty-four either remain in their own homes or live with an adult child. Elderly Swedes are less likely to share a house with their adult children than older Americans: 5 percent of the country's elderly population do so versus 15 percent in the United States.[74] For the relatively healthy, mobile, and active elderly, aging in place can be ideal, providing maximum privacy and comfort while allowing them to remain near part-time employment, volunteering opportunities, longtime neighbors, and community activities—that is, where social integration contributes so importantly to their health.[75] In fact, elderly Swedes are among Europe's leading volunteers with a participation rate of 17 percent.[76] Moreover, despite its generosity, the cost of Sweden's Home Help program is substantially lower than the alternative, which is the placement of elderly in nursing homes, where annual fees total approximately $70,000 per year.[77] However, the country's highly coordinated Home Help and health care network, which together enable aging in place, may sometimes inappropriately postpone an elderly person's transition to intermediate housing, such as an assisted living facility or more specialized housing that offers skilled nursing and memory care. These delays too often result, as former health and social affairs minister Ylva Johansson put it in 2006, too many "sick old people forced to stay at home too long."[78] Thus, Sweden's achievement of comprehensive programs to permit aging in place, which is the envy of many nations, also presents its own challenges, namely sustaining the elderly's social integration, which is critically important to strong health outcomes.

Indeed, a national AARP survey found that 82 percent of Americans would prefer to live out their lives in their current homes, even if they need assistance with the activities of daily living. Independence, privacy, and personal control thus appear to be values held in common in Sweden and the United States. Yet, despite the Americans' desire to age in place, services that assist them in doing so receive only 30 percent of federal long-term care expenditures; community-based social and nutrition programs that also support aging in place receive less than 1 percent.[79] The challenge is to create aging-friendly communities that encourage the building of social capital, provide home care, and facilitate health care services, all of which are important to strong health outcomes. One's socio-economic position, race, and ethnicity are important markers for elderly health in the United States, and they substantially affect the extent of one's access to age-friendly communities.

One-third of elderly African American women and one-half of Hispanic elderly women who live alone have annual incomes below the federal poverty rate ($12,490 for an individual in 2019). The absence of financial security can create insurmountable obstacles to overcoming disabling physical environments that are characterized by un-walkable neighborhoods and poor transport opportunities. The result is exclusion and the loss of social capital. Even the relatively well-off elderly are increasingly drawn away from aging in familiar neighborhoods and toward age-restricted "active senior living" communities where social and leisure-time activities permit social integration but health care access may be poor and bridging activities through intergenerational integration are rare.[80] The origins of age-restricted active senior communities are in the United States, the first being Sun City, Arizona, which opened in 1960, near Phoenix. As such, its creation and influence on the development of elderly housing in the United States is worthy of our attention.

Since the 1920s, Florida has been a winter haven for elderly Americans who could (or can) afford it. After the Second World War, many of the workers who had once escaped to Florida for a couple weeks of vacation during the winter decided to make the state their permanent residence in retirement. The growing wealth of America's elderly combined with air conditioning, better infrastructure, a warm albeit humid climate, and mosquito-killing DDT made Florida a popular retirement destination in the 1950s. But Florida's attraction, despite its boosters' best efforts to capitalize on an apocryphal story about a fountain of youth lying within its boundaries, remained its propinquity: in winter it was the closest warm place to New York and Chicago, and some very nice beaches came as a bonus.[81] Already home to age-restricted retiree communities by the late 1950s, Florida offered relaxation and leisure. But Del Webb, the founder of Sun City, envisioned something quite different: "an active new way of life."[82]

Webb built Sun City's houses so that they opened onto a golf course, an archery range, or lawn bowling field. He located a swimming pool and a wood shop at the community center. Webb called the early residents of his Sun City "pioneers," a term that encouraged their separation from the neighboring intergenerational communities. It implicitly designated areas outside Sun City as lands where lived "the other" people, younger ones. Property deeds required that at least one household occupant be at least fifty years of age or older; elderly married couples overwhelmingly occupied Sun City's two-bedroom, one-bathroom houses. Residency for children could only be granted for extraordinary reasons, but the social pressures against underage residency were enormous. Indeed, Webb granted permission to only two households where children could live— one for an air conditioning technician, the other for a primary-care physician. Both provided critical services to Sun City residents. Nevertheless, the school bus that entered the community to transport the families' children each day eventually provoked street protests. Soon the doctor and the AC repairman moved away.[83]

Despite the animosity of some residents toward intergenerational community living, the elderly of Sun City reported that their age segregation led to a remarkable comfort level among their fellows, which encouraged wide social integration. Anthropologists who have studied the phenomenon agree. The ease with which Sun City residents made friends appears to be linked to the absence of youth culture. As one resident remarked, "You don't feel old because you don't have the pressure of all those young people."[84] The community's strident age segregation created a "kind of communal conspiracy to continue living like human beings," free from comparisons with a younger generation with whom they felt increasingly alienated, especially as the anti–Vietnam War protests and youth counterculture grew in the 1960s and 1970s.[85] Yet "the other" outside of Sun City's walls was not just younger. It was also less white.

Sun City became a homogenous population of white middle-class and upper-middle-class elderly residents surrounded by more racially and ethnically diverse communities. The causes can be attributed to Webb and some residents who advocated a fortress attitude toward outsiders. From the beginning, Sun City's public relations manager Jerry Svendsen described moving to Sun City as "a Caucasian thing to do," and its vice president Tom Breen remarked that sales managers ought to explain to African American prospective buyers "what they are getting into because, let's face it, a Negro would be miserable in Sun City." In 1980, when Sun City had reached full capacity, African Americans constituted less than 1 percent of its forty-seven thousand residents compared to 4 percent in the greater Phoenix area.[86] More startling is the relative absence of Hispanic residents, even today. Only 3 percent of Sun City residents are Hispanic, while the surrounding Maricopa County is 31.3 percent Hispanic.[87]

Del Webb sold Sun City as a kind of fountain of youth where activities tailored to maintaining the health of the elderly residents abounded. But he did not intend it as a community where the elderly could healthfully age in place until their last days. Heavy reliance on automobile transportation constituted the most glaring deficit. An Arizona driver's license automatically expires at the age of sixty-five, requiring an in-person vision test for renewal and every five years thereafter, a process that eventually precludes renewal for the old-old (those over seventy-five). Sun City did not include assisted living facilities, which would have also improved residents' ability to age in place. Rather, Sun City and its many copies across the United States remain places where middle-class white elderly people can live independently until they must transition to more aging-friendly environments. Today Arizona alone, with a population of seven million, possesses some 105 Sun City–type age-restricted retirement communities, 8 with more than ten thousand residents and 3 with more than thirty thousand. Planning innovations pioneered at Sun City in 1960, such as placing a golf course at the center of the community and building hundreds of houses that open directly onto it, have also been imitated around the world.[88] But not in Sweden, at least not as a place where one can grow old only among other old people.

To the extent that Sweden had its own version of Del Webb, his name is Christer Jönsson. Inspired by Sun City, he created Victoria Park, a community in the Swedish city of Malmo that offers all the active-living facilities favored by Webb except a golf course. Jönsson marketed Victoria Park to the elderly, and it has become popular with them except for one crucial difference: Victoria Park also welcomes young families and has remained an intergenerational community.[89] The leading researchers on healthy aging, Andrew Scharlach and Amanda Lehning, advocate more "intergenerational programmes and social structures that promote meaningful roles for older adults and provide opportunities for frequent substantive interactions among persons of all ages, promoting development of significant bridging social capital across age cohorts."[90] The present US penchant for age-restricted communities is not likely to aid in this effort.

Elderly Health in the Age of Risk: 1990–Present

The 1970s marked a turning point in the economies of western Europe and the United States. Two oil price shocks (in 1973 and 1979) and competition from a rebuilt Japanese economy and the newly industrialized countries of South Korea, Taiwan, Singapore, and Hong Kong combined to challenge US economic dominance. Rising inflation and high unemployment—so-called stagflation—caused a recession like none that had struck the North Atlantic world since the end of the Second World War. By the late 1980s, as Swedish unemployment and inflation rose toward 10 percent and economic growth stalled, many observers predicted that Sweden's "people's home" (*folkhemmet*) could not survive. Payroll taxes stood at 36 percent, and the marginal income tax rate on high earners exceeded 80 percent; Sweden's overall tax burden was now the highest in the OECD. The nation had fallen from the fourth-richest OECD nation to the fourteenth. Between 1990 and 1993, the size of the Swedish economy *decreased* by 5 percent. A remarkable collapse of international competitiveness and the nation's standard of living were underway. Many Swedish and international observers blamed *folkhemmet*. The nation's welfare state, they said, had become too generous to afford.[91]

The ATP supplemental pension reform of 1960, which protected the elderly's financial security, emerged as a major culprit of the nation's economic woes. Slower economic growth and higher unemployment meant that earned pension rights were rising faster than wages and contributions. Also, ironically, better elderly health, made possible in part by the ATP supplemental pension, had raised Swedish life expectancy to among the highest in the world, but this very achievement exacerbated the fiscal strain on the economy. In order to maintain the solvency of the pension system, workers' contribution rates would have to rise from 19 to 24 percent by 2015 and then again to 30 percent by 2025.[92] Leaders across the political spectrum—five political parties representing 80 percent of voters—understood that such hikes were out of the question. With the central pillar of the "people's home" at stake, Sweden launched a series of social and economic reforms whose effectiveness amazed international observers. Indeed, economists at the International Labour Organization observed that the reforms resulted in "a revival and renaissance of the original Swedish model" that had been launched with the income tax–funded pension plan in 1913.[93]

A revamping of the pension system proved central to the reforms of the 1990s, taking advantage of the nation's gains in elderly health. First, reformers shifted the nation away from retirement funding that depended only on income tax revenues and current workers' contributions. Instead, Sweden adopted a *notional defined contribution* system based on individual retirement accounts, funded with a worker contribution of 16 percent of earnings. Benefit values from the new notional accounts were linked to lifetime earnings, economic growth, and demographic development. Together, these three components ensured the financial solvency of the system while encouraging (through its link to lifetime earnings) those who could to remain in the labor force. Second, in order to ensure equity between women and men and between socioeconomic groups, the new law recognized diverse forms of labor-market participation over the life course. For example, parents who leave the work force for childbearing and child rearing under the country's well-established paid family-leave programs (and who thereby bolster demographic growth and pension-system solvency) are not penalized for their absence from the active labor market in the calculation of lifetime earnings toward their pension benefits. Likewise, bouts of involuntary unemployment, often suffered by manual workers due to short-term disruptions in industrial production, do not suffer decreased lifetime earnings, nor do workers forced from employment due to sickness or disability. Third, the new system established an additional pension contribution of 2.5 percent that is invested in funds of the individual worker's choice and managed at low cost by a state pension administration. Because pension benefits in Sweden are now tied to economic and demographic strength through notional accounts, the new system is less vulnerable to insolvency than "pay-as-you-go" systems like US Social Security or those found elsewhere in Europe that rely directly on contributions from the active labor force.[94] The national economic rebound of the late 1990s, due in large measure to the pension and accompanying economic reforms, bolstered the foundation on which strong elderly health stands. The same wave of reforms also affected health care and long-term care services.

The Ädel Law of 1992 transformed the delivery of home care in Sweden. It transferred responsibilities for service delivery from the county councils to the nation's 289 municipalities. The Ädel Law also encouraged municipalities to contract private home-care agencies to help cover their caseloads. As a result, the proportion of private employment in the home-care sector rose from 2.5 to 13 percent, mostly due to the entry of international, for-profit home-care firms. These two changes might have been accomplished without altering access or quality of services. However, simultaneous cutbacks in hospital funding meant that more elderly were discharged back to their homes under new, accelerated protocols. Thus, even though funds for elderly care increased in real terms in the early 1990s, home-care providers faced greater numbers of acute-care and severe dementia cases that required more resources. As a result, access to simple ADL home-care services and preventive home health services fell. Research in the early 2000s indicated a growing disparity in access to such custodial home care according to socioeconomic class. High-income elderly forewent municipal home-care services, instead hiring care directly on the private market, while low-income retirees relied more heavily on family members or went without.[95]

More recent research indicates a correction of these trends and a renewed commitment to elderly care in order to attenuate disparities according to socioeconomic status and need. For example, since 2009, municipalities have been required to provide financial support to informal caregivers, including spouses, and the total volume of support provided by men and women is roughly equal. Equally important, longitudinal studies continue to indicate improvements in functional health in all new cohorts of seventy-year-olds; they are becoming more socially active in almost all aspects, including sexual activity but not church-going.[96]

The pension and elderly health care reforms of the mid-1990s played a major role in the revival of Sweden's "people's home" model. They maintained the elderly's financial security, access to health and long-term care, and social integration, which together play a crucial role in strong health outcomes. After 1996, Sweden's economic growth consistently exceeded both OECD and European Union averages. Annual household disposable income grew at 3 percent annually between 2006 and 2011. National debt fell from 80 percent of GDP in 1994 to 30 percent in 2012. Unemployment fell from 11 percent in 1997 to 5.5 percent in 2017. And Sweden's annual labor productivity growth now exceeds European, US, and OECD rates.[97] Little wonder that international observers, including the US business community took note. *Forbes* asked, "Is Sweden a bloated welfare state? Or a People's Republic of Entrepreneurs? The answer is it's a mixture of both. But the entrepreneurial part of the mix is rapidly gaining ascendancy."[98] Economists at the conservative Heritage Foundation judged, "Reforms in Sweden could be a model for U.S. lawmakers as they grapple with the problems of Social Security. . . . The same advantages would accrue to Americans and the American economy—but only if U.S. lawmakers learn the right lessons from what is happening in other nations."[99] Unfortunately, in recent decades the US elderly have experienced rising levels of financial insecurity, falling access to health care services, and a longstanding shortage of quality affordable long-term care.[100] These trends can be traced to the 1980s when the United States embraced a riskier form of retirement funding, which undermined the elderly's financial security and intensified health disparities.

The creation of Social Security in 1935 marked a turning point in old-age financial security in the United States. The program represents the nation's enduring commitment to support the elderly beyond their working years. Yet Social Security provides only a *basic pillar*. A system that ensures the widespread ability of the elderly to maintain a comparable standard of living (and thereby health outcomes) after leaving the labor force requires more than a basic pillar. During the Second World War, when the labor force was fully employed, the federal government imposed caps on wage increases to prevent runaway inflation that would have harmed the war effort. In order to retain their best employees and to preserve good labor relations, employers improved the private pension plans that were discussed earlier in this chapter. After the war, many in the white-collar and blue-collar middle classes relied on these pension plans as their *second pillar* of support. On top their Social Security benefits, they allowed retirees to maintain their standard of living after leaving the labor force. The 1950s to the 1980s were the heyday of these second-pillar supports, known as *defined-benefit* retirement plans.

Under a defined-benefit plan, the employee earns a specified retirement pension according to a predetermined formula based on annual earnings, years of service, and age. Contributions to the fund may be shared between employer and employee or paid entirely by one or the other. But in virtually all defined-benefit plans, the employer or labor union, as the case may be, assumes all risk to ensure that the pension fund will be able to provide the specified benefit to all eligible workers upon retirement. According to one of the foremost experts on the US retirement system, Sylvester Schieber, "If you sponsor a program to 'save' for workers' retirement security, along the way some saving has to be done. If you don't start early and stay at it, the bill is going to be mighty costly at the end."[101] Unfortunately, many corporate and union pension fund managers failed to heed this basic lesson.

Just as slowing world economic growth shook Sweden's pension system in the 1970s, so too the slowdown exposed the widespread underfunding of private and public pension plans in the United States. Congress duly stepped in, passing the Employee Retirement and Income Security Act (ERISA), which was meant to force employers to fund benefits as employees earned them. But it was too little too late. In the absence of more forceful state-led reforms, such as we saw in Sweden, many US firms discontinued their defined-benefit pensions. In their place, they latched on to another congressional innovation: tax legislation in 1978 that established 401(k) retirement plans. But in doing so, employers directly contradicted the intention of Congress. Congress intended 401(k) plans to function as a *third pillar* of the US retirement system, building on Social Security (basic pillar) and employer and union sponsored defined-benefit pensions (second pillar). Never were 401(k) plans meant to replace defined-benefit pensions because their approach to risk is fundamentally different. They are *defined-contribution* retirement plans.[102]

In contrast to a defined-benefit plan, a defined-contribution plan relies on employer or employee contributions (or both) to an individual investment account. Retirement benefits are based solely on the amount contributed and any income, expenses, gains, and losses. In short, all risk of building financial security for old age under a 401(k) plan is transferred from employer to worker because the employer is freed from investment choices. As a third and supplemental pillar—icing on the cake as it was intended—401(k) plans may have served well to supplement elderly financial security. Indeed, as we saw earlier, Sweden incorporated a comparable measure into its 1994 pension reform. But in Sweden only 2.5 percent of the 18.5 percent of total retirement savings are so allocated. In the United States, the 401(k) plan is replacing the second pillar of the nation's pension system: defined-benefit plans. In 1984, private defined-benefit plans had four times as many active workers as 401(k) plans, taking in three times the annual contributions. By 2007, the standings had nearly reversed: 401(k) plans had 2.6 times as many active participants as private defined-benefit plans and received approximately four times the contributions. Yet 401(k) plans remain voluntary, and many employers either do not offer them at all or offer no matching contributions.[103]

Meanwhile, in the public sector, many defined-benefit plans suffer from chronic underfunding. Moody's Investor Services estimates local and state government underfunding of their retirement pensions at $4.4 trillion, about 20 percent of the US GDP. Correction of the current shortfall would require tax hikes, the main source of state and local government funding, of about $32,000 per worker, an unlikely event in the foreseeable future.[104] In short, the second pillar of the US retirement system is either already gone or will soon disappear for most US workers. In fact, 401(k) plans were not designed to replace defined-benefit plans, and evidence already indicates that they are failing.[105]

A 2018 national survey found that 21 percent of working-age Americans have zero retirement savings, one-third have less than $5,000, and a third of baby boomers (those born between 1946 and 1964) have less than $25,000 dollars. The same survey indicated that fully 51 percent of respondents believed that it was either "not at all likely" or only "somewhat likely" that Social Security would be available when they retire.[106] The pessimism about the solvency of Social Security is overwrought and sometimes purposefully misrepresented by those who wish to abolish the program. The Social Security Administration actuaries foresee a shortfall to pay full benefits after 2034. After which, if no action is taken to replenish the trust fund, payments will fall to 77 percent of currently promised earned benefits and slip to 73 percent in seventy-five years. An increase in the Social Security payroll tax from its current 12.4 to 14.4 percent would be sufficient to allow the payment of full benefits for seventy-five years.[107] Whether US political leaders can reach a consensus on pension reform comparable to that of Sweden's leaders in the 1990s remains to be seen. The financial security and hence the health of the US elderly is at stake.

Our historical examination of the United States and Sweden has focused on the World Health Organization's social determinants of elderly health: financial security, social integration, and access to preventive and curative health services, including long-term care. History helps us understand why older Americans show poorer health outcomes than their Swedish counterparts. Such diverse outcomes are no accident. Sweden, like many European nations, has developed health and social services that explicitly recognize the role of the broad determinants of elderly health, changing services wherever and whenever possible to meet the changing local and global circumstances. This is made possible by a "determinants approach." That is to say, rather than perseverating on particular health deficits, diseases, or individual behaviors—although their recognition remains important—a determinants approach creates "societal conditions for good health on equal terms for the whole population." Since 2003, Sweden has been committed to a multi-sectoral strategy for improvement in the following "domains of objectives":

1. Participation and influence in society
2. Economic and social security
3. Secure and favorable conditions during childhood and adolescence
4. Healthier working life
5. Healthy and safe environments and products
6. A more health-promoting health service
7. Effective protection against communicable diseases
8. Safe sexuality and good reproductive health
9. Increased physical activity
10. Good eating habits and safe food
11. Reduced use of tobacco and alcohol, a society free from illicit drugs and doping, and reduction in the harmful effects of excessive gambling

Guided by these objectives, the Swedish National Institute of Public Health sets subgoals, coordinates local government policies, and measures progress in their attainment. Concern for the health of the elderly is readily apparent in goals one (social integration), two (financial security), and six (health care, including long-term care), whose history has been the focus of this chapter.

But equally important are factors that influence health earlier in the life course, such as a "healthier working life," under which private- and public-sector employers have committed to creating a labor market that is "more flexible and inclusive for individuals who have less than full working capacity." Similarly, local public transportation agencies recognize that "access to adequate transportation should be seen as an important part of people's economic and social security." A multi-sectoral determinants approach multiplies the effectiveness of efforts to ensure elderly people's financial security, social integration, and access to quality health and long-term care services.[108]

Conclusion

Beyond Medicine

Medicine is a social science and politics is nothing more than
medicine on a large scale.
—RUDOLF VIRCHOW, COLLECTED ESSAYS ON PUBLIC HEALTH
AND EPIDEMIOLOGY

The COVID-19 pandemic is just the latest of the great challenges to health systems around the world. Like the periods of industrialization, war, and economic crisis examined in this book, the pandemic makes clear that health care is but one of several influences that affect our potential to live a healthy life. We have seen that COVID-19 can sicken and kill many. But a much larger proportion of the population suffer from the pandemic's creation of financial insecurity, unemployment, precarious housing, hunger, and psychosocial stress, all of which have significant negative effects on health.

Our comparative analysis has taken up previous challenges to the health systems of France, Germany, Sweden, and the United States during similarly historic moments. When infant and maternal mortality were among the greatest threats to the health of families, the French responded with widespread milk pasteurization; universal maternal, infant and child care; public preschools; and parental leave. When urban industrial life and retirement insecurity emerged as significant threats to workers' health, Germany created social insurance to alleviate the risks of illness, disability, workplace accidents, and old age. The creation of works councils later facilitated the empowerment of German workers in their workplaces, an important psychosocial determinant of health. When Sweden faced an abrupt aging of its population because of emigration, the Swedes created the world's first income tax–funded universal pensions to assure the financial security of the elderly, which were later supplemented with effective home health services and universal long-term care.

Beginning in the nineteenth century, governments on both sides of the Atlantic became more involved in assuring the health of their populations. The vast social and physical changes wrought by industrialization and the growth of cities necessitated state-led public health measures to manage sanitation and control infectious disease. Yet the French, German, and Swedish governments played greater roles than the United States did in shaping the social determinants of health. The US government tended to defer to private-sector actors or to await state and municipal action. Even after the Supreme Court reinterpreted the Constitution to permit far-reaching federal action, the US government remained relatively meek compared to European states. It subsidized private actors, permitting them to shape the US health system in ways that later impeded the nation's ability to keep pace with health gains in the social democracies of France, Germany, and Sweden.

To be sure, social democratic health systems continue to face challenges of cost, equity, and quality. No system anywhere is immune to the challenges of aging populations and the rising cost of medical technologies. To these challenges we must add the disruptive forces of globalization, automation, and migration, which have undermined once sturdy foundations of employment and social peace in large regions of Europe and the United States. The hollowing out of once thriving industrial centers, from northern France to eastern Germany to the American upper Midwest, has led to unemployment, income stagnation, and despair, all of which are critical social determinants of health. Their connection to alcohol abuse, opioid addiction, and suicide is well documented.[1] Yet, of the four nations considered here, only the United States is suffering dramatic reversals in health outcomes, both relative and absolute. Indeed, in recent years, the life expectancy of Americans has fallen. In 1960, US life expectancy was 1.5 years *above* the average of other wealthy nations; now it is one year *below*, having fallen to 78.6 years.[2] The United States was also once a nation where families had a greater chance of escaping poverty in comparison to other wealthy nations. This is no longer the case. In fact, the decline in US socioeconomic mobility and stagnant incomes tracks the nation's relative decline in health outcomes.[3] When compared with European nations, the United States ranks among the lowest in social mobility. According to a major Brookings Institution study, "Starting at the bottom of the earnings ladder is more of a handicap [in the United States] than it is in other countries."[4] The plight of poor men is particularly problematic. Fully 42 percent of men born in 1958 into families in the bottom 20 percent of the income distribution remained there in 2006, while only between 25 and 30 percent of similarly disadvantaged men in Sweden, Denmark, the United Kingdom, and Norway remained at the bottom of their nations' income hierarchies. In fact, more poor men in these European nations achieved the rags-to-riches dream than their American counterparts. Between 11 and 14 percent of them climbed to the top quintiles of their country's income distribution versus only 8 percent in the United States. Both France and Germany also ranked above the United States in socioeconomic mobility. France's high-quality universal preschools and parental leave programs were identified as key drivers in the nation's performance.[5] We must remember that equity in the distribution of economic growth has important effects on a nation's social determinants of health. For example, between 1975 and 2005, US economic growth exceeded France's. But if the top 1 percent of households from both countries is excluded, we see that income growth for France's remaining 99 percent of households exceeded the income growth for the 99 percent of households in the United States.[6] Greater attention to more equitable distributions of wealth and income in European social democracies has benefited the health of their populations. Conversely, insufficient attention to household financial security in the United States has led to undue precarity and psychosocial stress, which help to explain the relatively poor state of Americans' health.

US Efforts to Improve Social Determinants of Health

This comparative history recognized the achievements of reformers who succeeded at decommodifying health without interrupting capitalist markets. They each improved a nation's social conditions in order to shield their people's health from unrestrained market forces. Germany's creation of social insurance in the 1880s set the rules by which the state, industrial employers, and their workers together insured themselves against the health risks of everyday life. In France, the 1930 grand bargain between the medical profession and the government enabled passage of the nation's public health insurance law while protecting private-practice medicine. In Sweden, the 1994 reforms of the nation's universal old-age pensions linked benefits to economic growth and channeled a portion of employee contributions into individual private accounts. This list should also include the 1935 creation in the United States of Social Security, which provides a modicum of financial security to elderly Americans even if health coverage was stripped from the original bill and long-term care remains woefully insufficient.

All of these reforms proved that dynamic states could protect the health of their citizenry in the face of large sociohistorical changes, whether it be a rapidly industrializing Germany, the Great Depression in France and the United States, or a Swedish economy wracked by increased global competition in the 1990s. These reforms stand in stark contrast to the sclerotic Soviet state of the 1980s that could not respond to the dramatic reversals in health outcomes. At the outset of this history, I posed the seemingly outrageous question whether the relative (and in some cases absolute) decline in Americans' health outcomes indicates an onset of the same kind of national fragility that contributed to the collapse of the Soviet Union in 1990. Certainly, the nearly decade-long political deadlock over health care reform since passage of the Affordable Care Act in 2010 signifies that the US government suffers from sclerosis. In the face of inaction, some health care providers and insurers have begun on their own to address what they call the social determinants of health for their neediest patients.

These efforts have primarily focused on food security, transportation, and housing. A Toledo, Ohio, health care system screens all its patients for nutritional needs and refers some of them to a "food pharmacy," which provides nutritious groceries without charge. A 2018 American Hospital Association study found that the system's food pharmacy clients used the emergency department 3 percent less, had 53 percent fewer hospital admissions, and visited their primary-care provider 4 percent more than comparable food-insecure patients who were not clients of the food pharmacy. Health care systems in Maryland, the District of Columbia, and Denver, troubled by costly no-show appointments for physical exams, have partnered with the ride-share companies Uber and Lyft to pay for patients who commonly miss medical appointments due to unreliable transportation. Their no-show rates have fallen dramatically as a result. A New York City health care system leases dozens of housing units and provides them on a short-term basis to frequent emergency room users, most of whom are homeless patients who suffer from chronic conditions. By avoiding multiple hospital readmissions and by freeing acute-care beds, the health care system reaped a 300 percent return on its housing investment.[7] Yet these programs, as beneficial as they are to some patients, do not address upstream social determinants where the impact is highest. They do not fundamentally alter "the physical and social environments in which people, grow, live, work, and age."[8] We must applaud a hospital that provides short-term housing, subsidizes groceries, or pays Uber rides for its patients in need. Yet that same hospital will not pay for the Uber ride of the same patients so they can get to work on time the next day, though no one denies that financial security is a fundamental social determinant of health and, in most cases, more important than a missed medical appointment.

The very existence of such programs indicates the need for state action. The government is uniquely capable of creating *public goods* that address social determinants that lie upstream, at the headwaters of health. A public good is a product that one individual can consume without reducing its availability to others and from which no one is deprived. Examples include mass transit systems, national defense, and public parks. Outlays to create them are often large, and their benefits are spread over the entire population and several generations. This makes the creation of public goods unattractive to private health care providers. Whether for-profit or nonprofit, their business model depends on the ability to measure a return on a specific investment.[9] What is more, to achieve their full potential, public goods require the exercise of state power.[10] For example, new bus and metro stops are far more effective if residents can safely walk to them, but only the state can condemn street-side private property to create sidewalks. At best, social determinants programs based in the health care industry can serve to ameliorate midstream causes of ill health. They provide short-term fixes for a limited number of patients but rarely create long-term, upstream solutions to poor health outcomes. At worst, such programs may serve to reinforce healthism—that is, a preoccupation with individual patients and the medicalization of their health conditions. Meeting individual patients' social needs represents a vertical integration of the health care sector, which may actually preserve social institutions that cause larger-scale ill health.[11]

Health care can improve individual quality of life and health outcomes. But our historical analysis of the French, German, and Swedish health systems shows that effective large-scale improvements in health outcomes

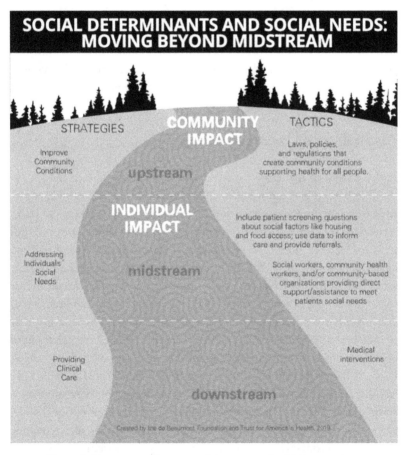

Figure 6. Upstream, midstream, and downstream health interventions.

Source: Brian Castrucci and John Auerbach, "Meeting Individual Social Needs Falls Short of Addressing Social Determinants of Health," *Health Affairs Blog*, January 16, 2019, https://www.healthaffairs.org/do/10.1377/hblog20190115.234942/full.

require the pairing of quality health care with investments in the structural conditions of life, from birth through the working years and old age. Health care-based social determinants programs fail to fundamentally transform the power relations that underlie poor US health outcomes.[12] As health foundation leaders John Auerbach and Brian Castrucci put it, focusing on the social needs of individual patients "can't raise the minimum wage, increase the availability of paid sick leave, or improve the quality of our educational systems. These are the systemic changes necessary to truly address the root causes of poor health."[13] Historical analysis of the development of social democracy in France, Germany, and Sweden corroborates their concern. In those three nations strong social safety nets, support for motherhood and families, occupational health, employees' power over their work, and assurances of financial security and long-term care in old age are key to the protection and maintenance of health.

The Health in All Policies Movement

Another front in the battle to improve US health outcomes is the Health in All Policies (HIAP) movement. Rather than relying on health care systems to attenuate the negative social determinants on individuals, HIAP recognizes head-on that transformational improvement requires political power. The term "Health in All Policies" emerged from Finland in 2006 during its presidency of the European Union, and it has spread widely since.[14] Health in All Policies is an "approach to public policies across sectors that systematically takes into account the health implications of decisions, seeks synergies, and avoids harmful health impacts, in order to improve population health and health equity."[15] These principles have been incorporated into European Union law and laws of many other nations, including the United States. For example, the 2010 Affordable Care Act distinctly includes HIAP guidelines to undergird its prevention provisions. New Zealand has embraced HIAP principles on a national scale, placing them on par with traditional economic priorities like economic growth and productivity in order to prioritize the citizenry's health and well-being as well as the environment.[16]

The HIAP movement has drawn critics who argue that asserting health into all public policy matters—economic, social, political, and cultural—

places health on par with time-honored principles such as private property, limited government, and freedom of belief. For example, if US firms were required to adopt German-style workplace health practices, which include greater employee influence over work, owners could argue that such a requirement violates their private property rights. If, in the interests of health, women were assured coverage of contraceptive and abortion services under their company health insurance plan, some private employers could claim a violation of their religious freedom to withhold such coverage. If increased regulation of firearms were deemed a public health imperative to save lives, some could challenge it as a violation of the Second Amendment to the Constitution. These are just a few poignant examples of how improvement in the social determinants of health can require transformational choices about the society in which we want to live. They also indicate the tremendous challenges faced by the HIAP movement.

The health impact assessment (HIA) plays a central role in the Health in All Policies approach. It informs policy makers and the greater public about how seemingly unrelated decisions outside the health field can affect health.[17] The HIA is modeled on the environmental impact assessment (EIA), a regulatory tool commonly used to evaluate the environmental effects of proposed projects. Similar to the EIA, the HIA is "a combination of procedures, methods, and tools that systematically judges the potential, and sometimes unintended effects of a policy, plan, programme or project on the health of a population and the distribution of those effects within the population." The HIA also "identifies appropriate actions to manage those effects."[18] Although the federal government does not require HIAs, they have long influenced decision making at the municipal and state levels. Twenty years ago, a HIA eased passage of San Francisco's living wage ordinance in 2000 by making transparent its positive health influences. More recently, a HIA exposed the negative impacts on climate change of plans to build a coal-fired power plant in Florida, which contributed to its cancellation. In Atlanta, the public transit authority employed a HIA when choosing among proposals for a major transit, trails, and parks project.[19] In 2010, California created a Health in All Policies Task Force, chaired by the state attorney general, which includes officers from eighteen state agencies whose activities possess influence over the social determinants of health.[20] All of these activities call attention to the importance of municipal and regional health system reforms and the potential benefits that the federal government's deployment of HIAs could foster.

Finding a Healthy Balance

In the introduction, we met Rudolf Virchow, the nineteenth-century Prussian physician who accused his own government of exacerbating the death toll of a typhus epidemic in Silesia. Virchow went on to found a "social medicine" movement that advocated better sanitation, public health, and preventive medicine. His followers pointed to epidemiological evidence that poor sanitation, inadequate housing, and unregulated industrial activities were the main causes of ill health and disease. Social medicine redefined what had previously been regarded as a *condition* of life, such as the occasional outbreaks of deadly disease, into a *problem* that could be solved through preventive measures. Its practitioners insisted that because human suffering was preventable, government authorities needed to act to mitigate it.[21] Indeed, governments on both sides of the Atlantic devoted substantial resources toward this end. In the 1860s, French emperor Louis Bonaparte razed major portions of Paris to replace open street sewers with a modern underground system; he also built massive aqueducts to bring cleaner freshwater from the Vannes River some two hundred miles away.[22] After a deadly cholera outbreak in Hamburg in the early 1890s, Germany's leading scientist, Robert Koch, arrived to chastise city leaders for their reckless disregard of health, a move that ended many political careers and led to the renovation of the city port, nearby housing, and the municipal water intake on the Elbe River.[23] Also in the 1890s, in the American Midwest, "sewer socialism" gained widespread support among Wisconsin voters who demanded better sanitation and public schools. Sewer socialists dominated Milwaukee politics and were part of Wisconsin's congressional delegation until the 1920s.[24] Yet soon thereafter social medicine was displaced by more narrowly focused biomedical and technological approaches.

Breakthroughs in germ theory and medical technologies, including antiseptics, anesthesia, pharmaceuticals, and diagnostic imaging, modified the very conception of health. The primacy of health promotion through attention to the broad social determinants of health—assuring potable water, improving sanitation and housing, regulating industrial toxic materials, ensuring financial security, et cetera—were overshadowed by individual curative measures. Community public health doctors became the poor cousins of the medical profession. By the late twentieth century, specialty providers and hospital systems had moved to the fore, propelled by biomedical and technological breakthroughs. Little wonder that today's health care system reflects a functional emphasis on individualized cure rather than public prevention, and medical specialization rather than primary care.[25]

The preeminent challenge of US social reform today is to create a balanced health system that can meet the challenges of the twenty-first century. Policies will need to simultaneously encourage continued progress in biomedical curative care, assure universal access to it, and enhance the social and physical environments that are imperative for a healthy life. Our comparative historical analysis reveals that purposeful state action in France, Germany, and Sweden helped to create balanced health systems that produce better population health outcomes than the United States.

In each of these European nations, a widespread perception of crisis proved critical to the success of government initiatives. The French saw the simultaneous stagnation of their population growth rate and German militarism as an existential threat to French civilization. This stimulated French state action to protect maternal and child health and encourage family formation. In Germany, a conservative ruling elite of aristocrats and industrialists recognized the real possibility that a socialist-led working class might replace them. In response, the German imperial state co-opted the leftist program through the creation of social insurance against the risks of everyday life, work, and old age. The Swedes likewise perceived a crisis born of emigration that had overwhelmed the wherewithal of their communities to care for the aged and infirm, who were left behind. They countered with the creation of an income tax–based system of old-age pensions. In each case, the crisis and the reaction to it constituted a critical juncture in health system creation that steered subsequent reforms, much in the way a climber of an old oak tree follows a chosen branch system to ascend higher and higher.

We must also bear in mind that the original ideological contexts of these critical junctures did not determine the nature of subsequent reforms. For example, through the creation of German social insurance in the 1880s, Bismarck meant to destroy the socialist movement. Yet this did not shield the institution he created from further reforms. Indeed, German social insurance eventually served as a founding pillar of German social democracy for which socialists played a lead role. Similarly, in the 1920s, most French employers who paid their workers extra if their wives remained at home with young children did so primarily because the allowance payments presented the most effective wage strategy at the time. Likewise, French pronatalist ideologues held decidedly retrograde views toward women's rights and equality, even in the context of their own era. Yet neither employers' unspoken pecuniary interest in the stay-at-home-mother allowance nor the reactionary sentiments behind the pronatalist movement determined the nature of subsequent reforms. Under the leadership of the French state, the concern for depopulation was transformed into a family-centered social democracy within a generation. By the same token, even the Swedes could not have predicted that their invention of income tax–funded old-age pensions in 1913 would lead through such tortuous reforms to emerge as the darling pension system of US conservative economists.[26] Swedish reformers sought to protect the financial security of their elderly and the solvency of their social democracy, which they achieved. The common thread here is the decommodification of health through a series of reforms, each embedded in its own particular national context.

Government's primary responsibility is to ensure the bodily security of the nation's citizenry. This is commonly understood to mean that the state must defend citizens from foreign armies. It should also mean that the government must provide reasonably safe social and physical environments for the living of healthy lives. Clearly, the decline in Americans' health outcomes compared to similar-income nations indicates a failure of the US government in this second and equally important responsibility. We should consider helpful approaches from abroad to improve Americans' health. A historical analysis can offer some guidance.

Like in France, Germany, and Sweden, the most important critical juncture in modern US health reform came in response to a national crisis. In the American case, it was the Great Depression of the 1930s. The 1935 Social Security Act promised financial relief to the nation's elderly in the form of pensions and unemployment insurance and jobs programs for idled workers. Yet the Social Security Act also served as the indispensable foundation on which subsequent health reforms have been built, right up to the present day. These include supplemental income for the disabled in the 1950s, Medicare and Medicaid in 1965, the 2003 addition of prescription drug coverage to Medicare, and the expansion of Medicaid under the 2010 Affordable Care Act. All were in varying ways amendments to the original Social Security Act of 1935. In this light, a clear pattern of progress emerges. Major US government action has proceeded in incremental fashion since the 1930s and has largely relied on a social-insurance approach. That is, workers pay for their social safety net benefits through paycheck deductions. However, as helpful as this method was in the creation of old-age pensions and the expansion of health coverage, flat-rate payroll deductions would ill serve our response to solve the twenty-first-century US health crisis. Payroll taxes are inherently regressive, exacting a greater burden on low- and middle-income earners. Rather than mitigate income inequality, itself a negative social determinant of health, payroll taxes exacerbate the problem.

Let us remember the economist Thomas Piketty's reflection that taxation is not merely a technical matter but "preeminently a political and philosophical issue, perhaps the most important of all political issues." As Piketty adds, "Without taxes, society has no common destiny."[27] Like Sweden, the United States possesses a progressive income tax that could be called into service to improve the nation's social determinants of health and replace regressive payroll taxes that currently fund many social benefits such as Social Security and Medicare. The first step is to return to the higher marginal income tax rates on high-income earners that were common in the 1960s, a decade of vibrant economic growth, in order to lower the tax burden on low- and middle-income earners. The United States could also collaborate with the European Union to craft a digital tax that would collect a share of the tech giants' windfall profits to improve education, health, and physical infrastructure. Second, the United States could incrementally expand the public health coverage that began in 1965 with Medicare and Medicaid, which was furthered by the 2010 Affordable Care Act. Medicare has demonstrated administrative efficiencies and outcomes-focused approaches, such as diagnosis-related group reimbursement, that are worthy of extension to the still uninsured sectors of the population. Third, we should elicit greater civic engagement in the revitalization of Americans' health. For example, if taxpayers could indicate preferences in how their money is expended—even non-binding ones—they might well choose to increase the funding of social programs.

Similar research shows that greater taxpayer agency could also dramatically reduce the "tax gap," which is the difference between total taxes owed and total taxes paid on time, some $458 billion annually.[28] If US income tax payers could direct some portion of their payment toward universal pre-K, paid sick leave and family leave, job training, and long-term care for the elderly, the federal income tax uptake might rise. Equally important, Congress could not ignore these potent referenda that signify Americans' recognition of our "common destiny" and their demands for access to a healthy life. The point here is not to identify any one policy initiative, a magic bullet, that would restore US population health to levels achieved by European social democracies. Rather, it is to urge experimentation with evidence-based, state-led approaches. Some approaches will prove more effective than others, but all should be judged by their outcomes, especially their health outcomes. In the end, the United States must find its own way, just as France, Germany, and Sweden have done since the nineteenth century.[29]

A promising sign is the current draft of *Healthy People 2030*, which will serve as a guiding framework for the US Department of Health and Human Services in the coming decade. It includes a hopeful sentence, one that does not appear in any previous *Healthy People* report: "Although much progress has been made, the United States lags behind other developed countries (such as other members of the Organisation for Economic Co-operation and Development) on key measures of health and well-being, including life expectancy, infant mortality, and obesity, despite spending the highest percentage of its gross domestic product on health."[30] This sentence marks a forthright recognition of where Americans might look for ideas to improve our health outcomes. It also indicates that reform of the nation's health care system alone will be insufficient to heal the nation.

The comparative historical evidence makes clear that government leaders can efficiently use the means at their disposal to shape and create markets—to make things happen that otherwise would not.[31] All three of the European health systems we have examined are embedded in market economies in which health has been recognized as an indispensable component of national prosperity. France, Germany, and Sweden are very different from each other, but they are bound by a common recognition that health is not only, or even primarily, an individual matter. It is a collective endeavor that is beyond medicine.

Notes

Introduction

1. Warren E. Buffet, "To the Shareholders of Berkshire Hathaway Inc.," March 1, 1993, https://www.berkshirehathaway.com/letters/1992.html.

2. For an excellent history on the making of social democracy, see Sheri Berman, *The Primacy of Politics: Social Democracy and the Making of Europe's Twentieth Century* (New York: Cambridge University Press, 2006).

3. "Paid Sick Leave: What Is Available to Workers?," US Bureau of Labor Statistics, https://www.bls.gov/ncs/ebs/factsheet/paid-sick-leave.htm.

4. Ben Zipperer and Josh Bivens, *Working Economics Blog*, Economic Policy Institute, April 16, 2020, "9.2 Million Workers Likely Lost Their Employer-Provided Health Insurance in the Last Four Weeks," https://www.epi.org/blog/9-2-million-workers-likely-lost-their-employer-provided-health-insurance-in-the-past-four-weeks.

5. Katie Johnston, "As More Grocery Store Workers Die, Employees Call for Better Protection," *Boston Globe*, April 7, 2020; " 'US Grocery Store Workers Need to Be Fairly Compensated': Protests at Amazon, Whole Foods Begin," *USA Today*, March 31, 2020; Letitia James, New York State Office of the Attorney General, "AG James' Statement on Firing of Amazon Worker Who Organized Walkout," March 30, 2020, press release.

6. Cour d'Appel de Versailles, Ministère de la Justice, "Communiqué relatif à l'affaire Amazon France Logistique c/ Union Syndicale Solidaire," April 24, 2020, press release; Alexandre Piquard and Betrand Bissuel, "Coronavirus: 'La mise en demeure d'Amazon confirme tout ce que nous disions,' " *Le Monde*, April 3, 2020.

7. US Agency for International Development, Project Predict, Reducing Pandemic Risk, Promoting Global Health, 2009, flyer, https://www.usaid.gov/sites/default/files/docu ments/1864/predict-global-flyer-508.pdf; Luca Lorenzoni and Francette Koechlin, *International Comparisons of Health Prices and Volumes: New Findings* (OECD, 2017).

8. Nicholas Kulish et al., "The U.S. Tried to Build a New Fleet of Ventilators; the Mission Failed," *New York Times*, March 29, 2020.

9. "Germany's Virus Response Shines Unforgiving Light on Britain," *Financial Times*, April 3, 2020.

10. "Deutschlands Coronavirus-Reaktion: Trunning von Fakt und Fiktion," *Deutschland Nachrichten*, April 7, 2020.

11. Keith Collins, "Coronavirus Testing Needs to Triple before the U.S. Can Reopen, Experts Say," *New York Times*, April 17, 2020; Katrin Bennhold, "With Broad, Random Tests for Antibodies, Germany Seeks Path out of Lockdown," *New York Times*, April 18, 2020.

12. White House, "Testing Blueprint: Opening up American Again," presidential briefing, April 27, 2020; "Trump Insists He Has 'Total' Authority to Supersede Governors," *New York Times*, April 13, 2020.

13. Kim Hjelmgard, "Swedish Official Anders Tegnell Says 'Herd Immunity' in Sweden Might Be a Few Weeks Away," *USA Today*, April 28, 2020.

14. Shikha Garg et al., "Hospitalization Rates and Characteristics of Patients Hospitalized with Laboratory-Confirmed Coronavirus Disease 2019—COVID-NET, 14 States, March 1–30, 2020," *Morbidity and Mortality Weekly Report* 69 (2020): 1–2.

15. Gretchen Livingston, "American Are Aging, but Not as Fast as People in Germany, Italy, and Japan," *Fact Tank* (Pew Research Center), May 21, 2015, https://www.pewresearch. org/fact-tank/2015/05/21/americans-are-aging-but-not-as-fast-as-people-in-germany-italy-and-japan.

16. Kenneth E. Thorpe et al., "Differences in Disease Prevalence as a Source of the U.S.-European Health Care Spending Gap," *Health Affairs* (October 2, 2007): 678–86.

17. National Research Council and Institute of Medicine, *U.S. Health in International Perspective: Shorter Lives, Poorer Health*, ed. Steven H. Woolf and Laudan Aron (Washington, DC: National Academies Press, 2013), 91.

18. David A. Kindig, "What Are Population Health Outcomes?," 2019, https://www. improvingpopulationhealth.org/blog/what-are-population-health-outcomes.html. See also David A. Kindig, "Understanding Population Health Terminology," *Milbank Quarterly* 85, no.1 (2007): 139–61; R. Gibson Parrish, "Measuring Population Health Outcomes," *Preventing Chronic Disease* 7, no. 4 (July 2010): 1–11; Robin Osborn et al., "Older Americans Were Sicker and Faced More Financial Barriers to Health Care than Counterparts in Other Countries," *Health Affairs* 36, no. 12 (2017): 1–10; "Health," OECD Better Life Index, http://www.oecdbetterlifeindex.org/topics/health.

19. "Global, Regional, and National Levels of Maternal Mortality, 1990–2015, a Systematic Analysis for the Global Burden of Disease Study 2015," *Lancet* 388 (October 2016): 1775–1812; "Pregnancy Mortality Surveillance System," Centers for Disease Control and Prevention, https://www.cdc.gov/reproductivehealth/maternalinfanthealth/pmss.html.

20. Anita Slomski, "Why Do Hundreds of U.S. Women Die Annually in Childbirth?," *Journal of the American Medical Association* 321, no. 13 (March 2019): 1239–1241.

21. "Maternal Mortality Ratio," World Bank Group, https://data.worldbank.org/indi cator/SH.STA.MMRT; Linda Villarosa, "Why America's Black Mothers and Babies Are in a Life-or-Death Crisis," *New York Times*, April 11, 2018.

22. Kathryn Strother Ratcliff, *The Social Determinants of Health: Looking Upstream* (Cambridge, UK: Polity Press, 2017), 2–6.

23. Michael Marmot and Jessica J. Allen, "Social Determinants of Health Equity," *American Journal of Public Health* 104, suppl. 4 (2014): S517–19.

24. "NNHHSTP Social Determinants of Health," Centers for Disease Control and Prevention, https://www.cdc.gov/nchhstp/socialdeterminants/faq.html.

25. Marmot and Allen, "Social Determinants of Health Equity," S517.

26. Thomas McKeown, *The Role of Medicine: Dream, Mirage or Nemesis?* (Princeton, NJ: Princeton University Press, 1980); Bernard Harris, "Commentary: 'The child Is the Father of the Man': The Relationship between Child Health and Adult Mortality in the 19th and 20th centuries," *International Journal of Epidemiology* 30 (August 1, 2001): 688–96; Robert F. Schoeni et al., eds., *Making Americans Healthier: Social and Economic Policy as Health Policy* (New York: Russell Sage Foundation, 2010), 6.

27. Robert Crawford, "Healthism and the Medicalization of Everyday Life," *International Journal of Health Services* 10, no. 3 (July 1980): 365–88.

28. Michel Foucault, *The Birth of the Clinic: An Archeology of Medical Perception,* trans. A.M. Sheridan (New York: Pantheon, 1973); Irving Zola, "Healthism and Disabling Medicalization," in *Disabling Professions (Ideas in Progress),* ed. Ivan Illich et al. (New York: Marion Boyars, 1977).

29. Peterson-KFF Health System Tracker, 2019, https://www.healthsystemtracker.org/chart-collection/health-spending-u-s-compare-countries/#item-start.

30. Martin A. Makary and Michael Daniel, "Medical Error—The Third Leading Cause of Death in the U.S.," *British Medical Journal,* 353i2139 (May 3, 2016), https://doi.org/10.1136/bmj.i2139.

31. CBS News Poll, Most Americans Favor a National Health Plan, October 15, 2019, https://www.cbsnews.com/news/2020-polls-national-health-care-plan-favored-by-most-americans-cbs-news-poll-finds; "Public's Assessment of the State of the U.S. Health Care System," Kaiser Health Poll Report, January–February 2004.

32. Steven A. Schroder, "We Can Do Better—Improving the Health of the American People," *New England Journal of Medicine,* 357, no. 12 (September 20, 2007): 1221–28.

33. Kyle Kinner and Cindy Pellegrini, "Expenditures on Public Health: Assessing Historical and Prospective Trends," *American Journal of Public Health* 99, no. 10 (October 2009): 1780–91; Samantha King, *Pink Ribbons Inc.: Breast Cancer and the Politics of Philanthropy* (Minneapolis: University of Minnesota Press, 2006).

34. Isaiah Berlin, "The Hedgehog and the Fox," *Classical Quarterly* 34 (1940): 26–29.

35. World Health Organization, "Social Determinants of Health," April 2019, https://www.who.int/social_determinants/sdh_definition/en; Ratcliff, *Social Determinants of Health,* 1–5.

36. Jill Quadagno, "Institutions, Interest Groups, and Ideology: An Agenda for the Sociology of Health Care Reform," *Journal of Health and Social Behavior* 51, no. 2 (June 2010):125–36.

37. F. Douglas Scutchfield and Alex F. Howard, "Moving on Upstream: The Role of Health Departments in Addressing Socioecologic Determinants of Disease," *American Journal of Preventative Medicine,* 40, no. 1S1 (January 2011): 80–83.

38. Jason Beckfield, Sigrun Olafsdottir, Benjamin Sosnaud, "Healthcare Systems in Comparative Perspective: Classification, Convergence, Institutions, Inequalities, and Five Missed Turns," *Annual Review of Sociology* 39 (June 2013): 127–46.

39. These include the US Agency for Healthcare Research and Quality, the Dartmouth College Center of Excellence, the National Bureau of Economic Research, and the Rand Center of Excellence. See Agency for Healthcare Research and Quality, "Defining Health Systems," https://www.ahrq.gov/chsp/chsp-reports/resources-for-understanding-health-systems/defining-health-systems.html.

40. Daniel Kim et al., "The Associations between US State and Local Social Spending, Income Inequality, and Individual All-Cause and Cause-Specific Mortality: The National Longitudinal Mortality Study," *Preventive Medicine* 84 (2016): 62–68; OECD, "Universal Health Coverage and Health Outcomes, Final Report," July 22, 2016, https://www.oecd.org/health/health-systems/Universal-Health-Coverage-and-Health-Outcomes-OECD-G7-Health-Ministerial-2016.pdf; James J. Heckman et al., "The Rate of Return to the HighScope Perry Preschool Program," *Journal of Public Economics* 94, nos. 1–2 (February 2010): 114–28; Jason Beckfield and Clare Bambra, "Shorter Lives in Stingier States: Social Policy Shortcomings Help Explain the U.S. Mortality Disadvantage," *Social Science & Medicine* 171 (2016): 30–38; Clare Bambra, "Cash versus Services: 'Worlds of Welfare' and the Decommodification of Cash Benefits and Health Care Services," *Journal of Social Policy* 34, no. 2 (April 2005) 195–213.

41. Jason Beckfield and Nancy Krieger, "Epi+demos+cracy: Linking Political Systems and Priorities to the Magnitude of Health Inequities—Evidence, Gaps, and a Research Agenda," *Epidemiologic Reviews* 31 (May 2009): 152–57.

42. Mariana Mazzucato, *The Entrepreneurial State* (New York: Public Affairs, 2015), 17.

43. Peter Baldwin, "Beyond Weak and Strong: Rethinking the State in Comparative Policy History," *Journal of Policy History* 17, no. 1 (January 2005): 12–33, quotation from 19.

44. Mazzucato, *Entrepreneurial State*, 15.

45. Health, United States, 2017 (Hyattsville, MD: US Dept. of Health and Human Services, 2018), https://www.cdc.gov/nchs/data/hus/hus17.pdf.

46. "Deaths in the United States, 2016," Centers for Disease Control and Prevention, http://blogs.cdc.gov/nchs-data-visualization/deaths-in-the-us.

47. C. E. A. Winslow, *The Evolution and Significance of the Modern Public Health Campaign* (New Haven: Yale University Press, 1923), 64–56.

48. National Research Council and Institute of Medicine, *U.S. Health in International Perspective*, 91.

49. When measuring the burden of disease on a population, epidemiologists employ a measure known has Disability Adjusted Life Years (DALYs). DALYs are a sum of lost healthy life years due to premature death plus the productive life years lost due to disabling health conditions. DALYs provide a more complete picture of a nation's health status than mortality rates because they show the burden of disease that arises from disabilities that may not ultimately cause death. See "Metrics: Disability Adjusted Life Year," World Health Organization, 2016, http://www.who.int/healthinfo/global_burden_disease/metrics_daly/en.

50. Cynthia Cox and Selena Gonzales, "The U.S. Has Highest Rate of Disease Burden among Comparable Countries, and the Gap Is Growing," Peterson-KFF Health System Tracker, July 7, 2015, http://www.healthsystemtracker.org/2015/07/the-u-s-has-highest-rate-of-disease-burden-among-comparable-countries-and-the-gap-is-growing.

51. Johan Galtung, "Violence, Peace, and Peace Research," *Journal of Peace Research* 6, no. 3 (1969): 167–91; Paul E. Farmer et al., "Structural Violence and Clinical Medicine," *PLOS Medicine* 3: no. 10 (October 2006): e449.

52. Philippe Bourgois, "Structural Vulnerability: Operationalizing the Concept to Address Health Disparities in Clinical Care," *Academic Medicine* 92, no. 3 (March 2017): 299–307; Janet Page-Reeves et al., "Health Disparity and Structural Violence: How Fear Undermines Health Among Immigrants at Risk for Diabetes," *Journal of Health Disparities Research and Practice* 6, no. 2 (Summer 2013): 30–47; James Quesada et al., "Structural Vulnerability and Health: Latino Migrant Laborers in the United States," *Medical Anthropology*, 30, no. 4 (July 2011): 339–62; S. D. Lane et al., "Structural Violence, Urban Food Markets, and Low Birth Weight," *Health Place* 14, no. 3 (September 2008): 415–23.

53. Bradley Sawyer and Daniel McDermott, "How Do Mortality Rates in the U.S. Compare to Other Countries?," Peterson-KFF Health System Tracker, 2019, https://www.

healthsystemtracker.org/chart-collection/mortality-rates-u-s-compare-countries/#item-start; Ramon Martinez et al., "Reflections on Modern Methods: Years of Life Lost Due to Premature Mortality—A Versatile and Comprehensive Measure for Monitoring Non-communicable Disease Mortality," *International Journal of Epidemiology* 48, no. 4 (August 2019): 1367–76.

54. Joseph Nye, "Who Caused the End of the Cold War," *Huffington Post*, May 25, 2011, https://www.huffingtonpost.com/joseph-nye/who-caused-the-end-of-the_b_350595.html.

55. "Director Admits CIA Fell Short in Predicting the Soviet Collapse," *New York Times*, May 21, 1992.

56. Christopher Davis and Murray Feshbach, *Rising Infant Mortality in the USSR in the 1970s*, Series P-95, 74 (Washington, DC: US Bureau of the Census, 1980).

57. Nick Eberstadt, "The Health Crisis in the USSR: A Review of Christopher Davis and Murray Feshbach, *Rising Infant Mortality in the USSR in the 1970s*, United States Bureau of the Census, Series P-95, No. 74, September 1980," *New York Review of Books*, February 19, 1981. See also Guillaume Vandenbroucke, "Russia's Demographic Problems Started before the Collapse of the USSR," *Economic Synopses* (Federal Reserve Bank of St. Louis), no. 4 (2016); *Vital and Health Statistics: Russian Federation and United States, Selected Years 1985–2000*, Vital and Health Statistics series 5, no. 11 (Hyattsville, MD: National Center for Health Statistics, 2003); Diane Rowland and Alexandre V. Telyukov, "Soviet Health Care From Two Perspectives," *Health Affairs* 10, no. 3 (Fall 1991): 71–86.

58. Nye, "Who Caused the End of the Cold War."

59. Eberstadt, "Health Crisis in the USSR."

60. *Health, United States, 2018* (Hyattsville, MD: US Dept. of Health and Human Services, 2019), https://www.cdc.gov/nchs/data/hus/hus18.pdf.

61. Holly Hedegaard et al., *Suicide Mortality in the United States, 1999–2017*, NCHS Data Brief 330 (Hyattsville, MD: US Department of Health and Human Services, Centers for Disease Control and Prevention, National Center for Health Statistics, 2018); Steven Stack, "Why Is Suicide on the Rise in the U.S.—but Falling in Most of Europe," *Conversation*, June 28, 2018, https://theconversation.com/why-is-suicide-on-the-rise-in-the-us-but-falling-in-most-of-europe-98366; Shekhar Saxena et al., *Preventing Suicide: A Global Imperative* (Geneva: World Health Organization, 2014).

62. Mercedes R. Carnethon et al., "Cardiovascular Health in African Americans: A Scientific Statement from the American Heart Association," *Circulation* 136, no. 21 (November 21, 2017), 10.1161/CIR.0000000000000534.

63. "Disparities," Indian Health Service, October 2019, https://www.ihs.gov/newsroom/factsheets/disparities.

64. Anne Case and Angus Deaton, "Rising Morbidity and Mortality in Midlife among White Non-Hispanic Americans in the 21st Century," *Proceedings of the National Academy of Sciences* 112, no. 49 (December 2015):15078–83.

65. Jason Beckfield and Katherine Morris, "Health," in "State of the Union: The Equality and Poverty Report 2016," special issue of *Pathways* (Stanford Center of Poverty and Inequality), 2016, 58–64, https://inequality.stanford.edu/sites/default/files/Pathways-SOTU-2016.pdf; Richard Wilkinson and Kate Pickett, *The Spirit Level: Why Greater Equality Makes Societies Stronger* (London: Bloomsbury, 2009).

66. Georges Lefebvre, *La grande peur de 1789: Suivi de Les Foules révolutionnaires* (Paris: Armand Colin, 2014); Georges Rudé, "Prices, Wages and Popular Movements in Paris during the French Revolution," *Economic History Review* 6, no. 3 (April 1954): 246–67.

67. Thomas Piketty, *Capital in the Twenty-First Century* (Cambridge, MA: Harvard University Press, 2017), Kindle ed., 630.

68. Dana Simmons, *Vital Minimum: Need, Science, and Politics in Modern France* (Chicago, University of Chicago Press, 2015).

69. Marc Bloch, "Pour une histoire comparée des sicítéts européenes," *Revue de Synthèse Historique* 46 (1928): 15–50.

70. Daniel T. Rogers, *Atlantic Crossings: Social Politics in a Progressive Age* (Cambridge, MA: Harvard University Press, 1998), 3.

71. John W. Ward and Christian Warren, eds., *Silent Victories: The History and Practice of Public Health in Twentieth-Century America* (New York: Oxford University Press, 2007); Sandro Galea, *Macrosocial Determinants of Population Health* (New York: Springer, 2007); Colin Woodard, *American Nations: A History of the Eleven Rival Regional Cultures of North America* (New York: Penguin, 2001).

72. Margaret Levi, "A Model, a Method, and a Map: Rational Choice in Comparative Historical Analysis," in *Comparative Politics: Rationality, Culture, and Structure*, ed. Mark I. Lichbach and Alan S. Zuckerman (Cambridge, UK: Cambridge University Press, 1997), as cited by Paul Pierson, "Increasing Returns, Path Dependence and the Study of Politics," *American Political Science Review* 94, no. 2 (June 2000): 252. See also Paul Pierson, *Politics in Time: History, Institutions, and Social Analysis* (Princeton, NJ: Princeton University Press, 2004).

73. National Research Council and Institute of Medicine, *U.S. Health in International Perspective*, 287.

74. Mervyn Susser and Ezra Susser, foreword to *A Life Course Approach to Chronic Disease and Epidemiology*, ed. Diana Kuh and Yoav Ben-Schlomo (New York: Oxford University Press, 2004), vii.

75. Introduction to Kuh and Ben-Schlomo, *Life Course Approach to Chronic Disease*, 5; George Davey Smith and John Lynch, "Life Course Approaches to Socio-economic Differentials in Health," in Kuh and Ben-Schlomo, *Life Course Approach to Chronic Disease*, 107.

76. Barry Bogin, "Human Growth and Development from an Evolutionary Perspective," and C. J. K. Henry, "Early Environmental and Later Nutritional Needs," in *Long-Term Consequences of Early Environment: Growth, Development, and the Lifespan Developmental Perspectives*, ed. C. J. K. Henry and S. J. Ulijaszek (Cambridge, UK: Cambridge University Press, 1996), 7–21, 124–38.

77. "Infant Mortality Rates," OECD, https://data.oecd.org/healthstat/infant-mortality-rates.htm.

78. Clare Bambra, *Work, Worklessness, and the Political Economy of Health* (Oxford: Oxford University Press, 2011).

79. "*Global AgeWatch Index 2015*," HelpAge International, 2015, http://www.helpage.org/global-agewatch.

80. *World Report on Ageing and Health* (Geneva: World Health Organization, 2015).

81. Erwin H. Ackerknecht, *Rudolf Virchow: Doctor, Statesman, Anthropologist* (Madison: University of Wisconsin Press, 1953), 123–32.

82. Rudolf Virchow, "Report on the Typhus Epidemic in Upper Silesia," in *Collected Essays in Public Health and Epidemiology*, ed. L. J. Rather (Sagamore Beach, MA: Watson Publishing, 1985), 18.

83. Myron Schultz, "Rudolph Virchow, 1821–1902)," *Emerging Infectious Diseases* 14, no. 9 (September 2008): 1480–81, http://www.ncbi.nlm.nih.gov/pmc/articles/PMC2603088/#!po=83.3333.

84. J. P. Mackenbach, "Politics Is Nothing but Medicine on a Larger Scale: Reflections on Public Health's Biggest Idea," *Journal of Epidemiology and Community Health* 63, no. 3 (March 2009): 181–84; Michael Marmot, "The Influence of Income on Health: Views of an Epidemiologist," *Health Affairs* 21, no. 2 (March/April 2002), 31–46.

1. Infant and Child Health in the United States and France

1. Carlo A. Corsini and Pier Paulo Viazzo, eds., *The Decline of Infant Mortality in Europe, 1800–1950, Four National Case Studies* (Florence: UNICEF International Child Developmental Centre and Istituto degli Innocenti, 1993), 7, https://www.unicef-irc.org/pub lications/pdf/hisper_decline_infantmortality_low.pdf.

2. National Research Council and Institute of Medicine, *U.S. Health in International Perspective: Shorter Lives, Poorer Health*, ed. Steven H. Woolf and Laudan Aron (Washington, DC: National Academies Press, 2013), 61. The World Health Organization defines the perinatal period as starting with the twenty-eighth week of pregnancy and ending one week after birth. US health providers generally consider the perinatal period to commence in the twenty-second week of pregnancy and end one week after birth. The French Health Ministry notes that the perinatal period may include the full period of gestation and include the entire neonatal period, which begins with birth and ends four weeks later.

3. Similar-income nations here are derived from child poverty rates from members of the Organisation for Economic Cooperation and Development. "OECD Family Database," http://www.oecd.org/els/family/database.htm; *Doing Better for Children* (OECD, 2019), Chart CO2.2.2.A, https://www.oecd.org/els/family/doingbetterforchildren.htm.

4. Nicholas Kassebaum, et al., "Global, Regional, and National Levels of Maternal Mortality, 1990–2015: A Systematic Analysis for the Global Burden of Disease Study 2015," *Lancet*, 388, no. 10053 (October 2016): 1775–1812; "Pregnancy Mortality Surveillance System," Centers for Disease Control and Prevention, 2019, https://www.cdc.gov/reproductive health/maternalinfanthealth/pmss.html.

5. Ashish P. Thakrar et al., "Child Mortality in the U.S. and 19 OECD Comparator Nations: A 50-Year Time Trend Analysis," *Health Affairs* 37, no. 1 (January 2018): 140–49.

6. Marian F. MacDorman and T. J. Matthews, "Understanding Racial and Ethnic Disparities in U.S. Infant Mortality Rates," *NCHS Data Brief* (National Center for Health Statistics) 74 (September 2011): 1, https://www.cdc.gov/nchs/data/databriefs/db74.pdf; The World Bank, "International Migrant Stock (% of Population)," 2008 revision, https://data.world bank.org/indicator/SM.POP.TOTL.ZS.

7. T. J. Mathews and M. MacDorman, "Infant Mortality Statistics from the 2004 Period Linked Birth/Infant Death Data Set," *National Vital Health Statistics Report 55*, no. 14 (2007): 7–9.

8. National Research Council and Institute of Medicine, *U.S. Health in International Perspective*, 67–68.

9. *Journal Officiel*, February 2, 1882, Rapport concernant l'application de la loi du 23 décembre 1874, as cited by Alain Norvez, *De la naissance à l'école: santé, modes de garde et préscolarité dans la France contemporaine* (Paris: Institut National d'Études Démographiques et Presses Universitaires de France, 1990), 14. Here and in the following, all English-language quotations from French sources are the author's translations.

10. Catherine Rollet-Echalier, *La Politique à l'égard de la petite enfance sous la IIIe République*, Travaux et Documents Cahier 127 (Paris: Institut National d'Études Démographiques et Presses Universitaires de France, 1990), 282–84; Catherine Rollet, "The Fight against Infant Mortality in the Past: An International Comparison," in *Infant and Child Mortality in the Past*, ed. Alain Bideau et al. (London: Clarendon, 1997), 43–44.

11. Norvez, *De la naissance à l'école*, 14; Jack Ellis, *The Physician-Legislators of France: Medicine and Politics in the Early Third Republic, 1870–1914* (Cambridge, UK: Cambridge University Press, 1990), 220–23.

12. Elizabeth Fee, "Public Health and the State," in *The History of Public Health and the Modern State*, ed. Dorothy Porter (Amsterdam: Rodopi, 1994), 233.

13. Ibid.

14. Ibid., 241.

15. Frederick L. Hoffman, *Race Traits of the American Negro*, vol. 11, nos. 1–3 (New York: American Economic Association, 1896), 95. Italics in original.

16. Richard A. Meckel, *Save the Babies: American Public Health Reform and the Prevention of Infant Mortality, 1850–1929* (Baltimore: Johns Hopkins University Press, 1990), 131–33.

17. Paul V. Dutton, "Battle for Control of Social Welfare: Workers vs. Employers," chap. 3 in *Origins of the French Welfare State: The Struggle for Social Reform in France, 1914–1947* (New York: Cambridge University Press, 2002); Bruno Valat, *Histoire de la Sécurité Sociale: L'État, l'institution de la santé* (Paris: Economica, 2001); Henri Hatzfeld, *Du Paupérisme à la sécurité sociale: 1850–1940* (Nancy: Presses Universitaires de Nancy, 1989); Dominique Ceccaldi, *Histoire des prestations familiales en France* (Paris: Union Nationale des Caisses d'Allocations Familiales, 1957).

18. Catherine Rollet, "La construction d'une culture international autour de l'enfant," in *Comment peut-on être socio-anthropologue? Autour d'Alain Girard* (Paris: Harmattan, 2000), 149. For an overview of paternalist social welfare policies in France and elsewhere, see Kathryn Kish Sklar, "A Call for Comparisons," *American Historical Review* 95, no. 4 (October 1990): 1109–14.

19. Paul Strauss, *Dépopulation et puericulture* (Paris: L. Maretheux, 1901), 4.

20. Ibid., 5, 79, 301.

21. Charles Candiotti and Marcel Moine, *La Mortalité de l'enfant de première année* (Paris: Ballière et fils, 1948), 46.

22. Pierre Budin, *The Nursling: The Feeding and Hygiene of Premature and Full-Term Infants*, trans. William J. Maloney (London: Caxton Publishing, 1907), 151.

23. "Milk station" is a functional translation of *goutte de lait*. The literal translation is "drop of milk." Some public health advocates outside of France—in Canada, for example—who adapted the practice for their own countries also imported the French term, calling their dispensaries "*Gouttes de Lait.*"

24. Catherine Rollet, "La Santé et la protection de l'enfant vues à travers les congrès internationaux (1880–1920)," *Annales de démographie historique* 101 (January 2001), 97–116, 104–5.

25. Budin, *Nursling*, 156, 148.

26. Catherine Rollet, "La Santé et la protection de l'enfant," 103.

27. Ibid., 103–4.

28. Thomas Morgan Rotch, *Pediatrics: The Hygienic and Medical Treatment of Children* (Philadelphia: Lippincott, 1896), 159.

29. Ibid., 214.

30. Meckel, *Save the Babies*, 57–58.

31. Ibid., 55–59.

32. "Dr. Abraham Jacobi Dies Suddenly at 89," *New York Times*, July 12, 1912; Julie Miller, *Abandoned: Foundlings in Nineteenth-Century New York City* (New York: New York University Press, 2008), 176–80.

33. It must be remembered that knowledge of vitamins remained theoretical until the 1920s, and empirical studies of their hardiness in the face of pasteurization would not be fully understood until even later. See Richard D. Semba, "The Discovery of Vitamins," *International Journal of Vitamins and Nutritional Research* 82, no. 5 (October 2012): 310–15.

34. Meckel, *Save the Babies*, 77–81.

35. Robert V. Tauxe and Emilio J. Estaban, "Advances in Food Safety to Prevent Foodborne Diseases in the United States," in *Silent Victories: The History and Practice of Public*

Health in Twentieth-Century America, ed. John W. Ward and Christian Warren (New York: Oxford University Press, 2007), 25.

36. Charles E. North, *Report of Rochester Milk Survey by the Committee on Public Safety of the Common Council* (New York: City of Rochester, 1919), 189–203.

37. The theory of demographic transition posits that the relationship between industrialization and fertility is inverse: industrialization raises living standards and stimulates a general aspiration toward increasingly greater degrees of comfort, which, in turn, promotes a limitation on childbearing. This theory is opposed by Malthusian theory, which states that economic development stimulates fertility, increases the demand for work, and encourages marriage and family formation. Conformity with both theories has been widely observed. During the initial stages of industrialization, countries have witnessed rapid rises in fertility; subsequent decades brought a demographic transition. See Jean-Claude Chesnais, *The Demographic Transition: Stages, Patterns, and Economic Implications* (Oxford, UK: Clarendon Press, 1992).

38. Cheryl Koos, "Gender, Anti-Individualism, and Nationalism: The Alliance Nationale and the Pronatalist Backlash against the Femme Moderne, 1933–1940," *French Historical Studies* 19, no. 3 (Spring 1996): 699–723. Alisa Klaus, *Every Child a Lion: The Origins of Maternal and Infant Health Policy in the United States and France, 1890–1920* (Ithaca, NY: Cornell University Press, 1993), 5–6.

39. "Rerum Novarum," Claudia Carlen, ed., *The Papal Encyclicals, 1878–1903* (Wilmington, NC: McGrath, 1981), 241–61.

40. William Oualid and Charles Picquenard, *Salaires et tarifs, conventions collectives et grèves: la politique du Ministère de l'Armement et du Ministère du Travail* (Paris: Presses Universitaires de France, 1928), 105–8. Allowances struck a hard blow to women workers who were fighting for equal pay for equal work. Family allowances were generally only paid to those who held the status of *chef de famille*, a distinction denied to women as long as they were married, even if their husbands worked in a profession where allowances were not available. Some industrialists paid allowances to abandoned women who could demonstrate de facto custodianship of children with a letter from their neighborhood police. Male heads of household were simply required to provide a registered birth certificate for each eligible child.

41. Dutton, "An Industrial Model of Family Welfare," chap. 1 in *Origins of the French Welfare State*.

42. Susan Pedersen, "Catholicism, Feminism, and the Politics of the Family during the late Third Republic," in *Mothers of a New World: Maternalist Politics and the Origins of Welfare States*, ed. Seth Koven and Sonya Michel (New York: Routledge, 1993), 246–76. See especially note 270n6.

43. Eve Baudouin, *La mère au travail et le retour au foyer* (Paris: Librarie Bloud et Gay, 1931), 24, 25–27. See also Eve Baudouin, "Pour la mère au foyer," *Chronique sociale de France*, March 15, 1939, 199–211.

44. *Journal Officiel de la République Francaise*, Documents parlementaires, Chambre, March 28, 1935, annexe no. 5193, 777. See also Conseil Supérieur de la Natalité, Communications 1934, no. 3, Section permanente, *procès-verbaux*, January 16, 1934, 16–18.

45. *Journal Officiel de la République Francaise*, Documents parlementaires, Chambre, April 27, 1937, annexe no. 2276, remarks of Deputy Reille-Souille, 515. See also legislation by Henri Becquart, *Journal Officiel de la République Francaise*, Documents parlementaires, Chambre, June 6, 1936, annexe no. 176, 222.

46. *Journal Officiel de la République Francaise*, Documents parlementaires, Chambre, April 2, 1939, Règlement d'administration publique, 4396.

47. Theda Skocpol, *Protecting Soldiers and Mothers: The Political Origins of Social Policy in the United States* (Cambridge, MA: Harvard University Press, 1992), 322.

48. Quoted in Mark Leff, "Consensus for Reform: The Mothers' Pension Movement in the Progressive Era," *Social Service Review* 47, no. 3 (September 1973): 399.

49. *Report of the Proceedings of the Thirty-First Annual Convention of the American Federation of Labor, Atlanta, GA, November 13–25, 1911* (Law Reporter Printing, 1911), 357–58.

50. Skocpol, *Protecting Soldiers and Mothers*, 424; Peter V. Fishback and Shawn Everett Kantor, "The Adoption of Workers' Compensation, 1900–1930," National Bureau of Economic Research Working Paper 5840 (November 1996), 1–3, 49.

51. Skocpol, "An Unusual Victory for Public Benefits: The 'Wildfire Spread' of Mothers' Pensions," chap. 8 in *Protecting Soldiers and Mothers*.

52. Ferdinand Éduoard Buisson, "*Crèches, historique,*" *Nouveau dictionnaire de pédagogie*, l'edition électronique, Institut Français de l'Éducation, http://www.inrp.fr/edition-electro nique/lodel/dictionnaire-ferdinand-buisson/document.php?id=2488.

53. Catherine Rollet, "Évolution des mode de garde de l'enfant," Paper presented at the Comité National de l'Enfance, Paris, December 3, 2009.

54. Eugen Weber, "Civilizing in Earnest," chap. 18 in *Peasants into Frenchmen: The Modernization of Rural France, 1870–1914* (Stanford, CA: Stanford University Press, 1976).

55. Inspection Générale de l'Éducation Nationale, Inspection Générale de l'Administration de l'Éducation Nationale et de la recherche, *L'École Maternelle*, report no. 2011-108 (Paris: Ministère de l'Éducation Nationale, de la Jeunesse, et de la Vie Associative, October 2011), 14–23, 37–44, 64–71.

56. Emily Cahan, *Past Caring: A History of U.S. Preschool Care and Education for the Poor, 1820–1965* (New York: National Center for Children in Poverty and Columbia University Mailman School of Public Health, 1989); Barbara Beatty, *Preschool Education in America: The Culture of Young Children from the Colonial Era to the Present* (New Haven, CT: Yale University Press, 1995); "Early Childhood Education Act," K12 Academics, https://www. k12academics.com/Federal%20Education%20Legislation/early-childhood-education-act.

57. Molly Ladd-Taylor, "Federal Help for Mothers: The Rise and Fall of the Sheppard-Towner Act in the 1920s," in *Gendered Domains: Rethinking Public and Private in Women's History*, ed. Dorothy O. Helly and Susan M. Reverby (Ithaca, NY: Cornell University Press), 1992, 217–18.

58. Meckel, *Save the Babies*, 212.

59. Louis J. Covotsos, "Child Welfare and Social Progress: The United States Children's Bureau, 1912–1935," PhD diss., University of Chicago, Dept. of History, 1976, 123, quoted in Skocpol, *Protecting Soldiers and Mothers*, 500.

60. Kimberly Johnson, *Governing the American State: Congress and the New Federalism, 1877–1929* (Princeton, NJ: Princeton University Press, 2007), 148.

61. Jessamine S. Whitney and the US Children's Bureau, *Infant Mortality: Results of a Field Study in New Bedford, Mass. Based on Births in One Year* (Washington, DC: US Department of Labor, 1920); Kriste Lindenmeyer, "Saving Mothers and Babies: Designing and Implementing a National Maternity and Infancy Act, 1918–30," chap. 4 in *"A Right to Childhood": The U.S. Children's Bureau and Child Welfare, 1912–1946* (Champaign: University of Illinois Press, 1997).

62. Johnson, *Governing the American State*, 151–54; Karen Davis and Cathy Schoen, *Health and the War on Poverty: A Ten-Year Appraisal* (Washington, DC: Brookings Institution, 1978) 120–22.

63. Skocpol, *Protecting Soldiers and Mothers*, 505; Johnson, *Governing the American State*, 48–49.

64. John Duffy, *The Sanitarians: A History of American Public Health* (Champaign: University of Illinois Press, 1990), 249.

65. "Minutes of the Seventy-Third Annual Session of the American Medical Association, St. Louis, May 22–26, 1922," *Journal of the American Medical Association* 78 (1922): 1715.

66. Alice Sardell, *The U.S. Experiment in Social Medicine: The Community Health Center Program, 1965–1986* (Pittsburgh: University of Pittsburgh Press, 1988), 26.

67. Covotsos, "Child Welfare and Social Progress," quoted in Skocpol, *Protecting Soldiers and Mothers*, 517.

68. Paul V. Dutton, *Differential Diagnoses: A History of Health Care Problems and Solutions in the United States and France* (Ithaca, NY: Cornell University Press, 2007), 79–80.

69. Paul Cibrie, *Syndicalisme médical* (Paris: Confédération des Syndicats Médicaux Français, 1954), 70.

70. *Journal Officiel de la République Française*, Ordonnance no. 45-2454, October 19, 1945. See esp. articles 10, 12–13.

71. Norvez, *De la naissance à l'école*, 77.

72. Charles de Gaulle, *Memoirs d'espoir: L'esprit de la Vème République* (Paris: Plon, 1970), 70.

73. Alain Contrepois, *Les Jeunes enfants et la crèche: un histoire* (Paris: Editions des Archives Contemporaines, 2006), 78–94.

74. Norvez, *De la naissance à l'école*, 79–87, 91–110, 137–59.

75. The *carnet de santé* was hardly a new document to French families. In the late nineteenth century, the physician Jean-Baptiste Fonssagrives published a notebook intended for mothers and attending medical providers to record their observations about a child's health and growth. Thereafter, medical and public health officials openly debated whether use of the *carnet* should be compulsory. A decisive break came in 1939 when the city of Bordeaux introduced a version in which only medical providers could record actions and observations, marking a milestone in the medicalization of infant and child health care that had been underway for some fifty years. Bordeaux's "doctor's only" version soon became the standard throughout France. See Catherine Rollet, "History of the Health Notebook in France: A Stake for Mothers, Doctors and State," in *Dynamis: Acta Hispanica ad Medicinae Scientiarumque Historiam Illustrandam* 23 (2003): 143–66.

76. Norvez, *De la naissance à l'école*, 91–94; "Congé maternité d'une salariée du secteur privé," République Française, Service-Public.fr ("Le site officiel de l'administration française"), https://www.service-public.fr/particuliers/vosdroits/F2265.

77. Marie-Laure Cadart, "L'Enfant et la PMI, d'hier à aujourd'hui: Entre medical, social et politique," *Informations sociales* 4, no. 140 (2007): 52–63.

78. "Congé maternité d'une salariée du secteur privé."

79. "Total Fertility Rate," World Factbook, Central Intelligence Agency, https://www.cia.gov/library/publications/the-world-factbook/fields/356.html.

80. Lisa F. Berman and Maria Melchoir, "The Shape of Things to Come: How Social Policy Impacts Social Integration and Family Structure to Produce Population Health," in *Social Inequalities in Health*, ed. Johannes Siegrist and Michael Marmot (New York: Oxford University Press, 2006), 67.

81. Milton Kotelchuck, "Safe Mothers, Healthy Babies: Reproductive Health in the Twentieth Century," in Ward and Warren, *Silent Victories*, 114.

82. Jennifer Klein, *For All These Rights, Business, Labor, and the Shaping of America's Public-Private Welfare State* (Princeton, NJ: Princeton University Press, 2003), 166–69.

83. *Journal of the American Medical Association* 127, no. 2 (January 13, 1945): 102.

84. Stephen P. Strickland, *Politics, Science, and Dread Disease: A Short History of United States Medical Research Policy* (Cambridge, MA: Harvard University Press, 1972), 50.

85. Elizabeth Fee, "Public Health and the State," 250–54.

86. Anne R. Somers and Herman M. Somers, "Health Insurance: Are Cost and Quality Controls Necessary?" *Industrial and Labor Relations Review* 13, no. 4 (July 1960): 581; *Journal of the American Medical Association* 179, no. 13 (March 31, 1962): 17.

87. For a comprehensive account of Medicaid's creation, see Robert Stevens and Rosemary Stevens, *Welfare Medicine in America: A Case Study of Medicaid* (New York: Transaction, 2003).

88. Daniel R. Levinson and US Department of Health and Human Services, Office of the Inspector General, *Most Medicaid Children in Nine States Are Not Receiving All Required Preventive Screening Services*, OEI 05–08–00520 (Washington, DC: US Department of Health and Human Services, Office of the Inspector General, 2010); US Government Accountability Office, *Medicaid Preventive Services: Concerted Efforts Needed to Ensure Beneficiaries Receive Services*, GAO 09–578 (Washington, DC: US Government Accountability Office, 2009).

89. Milton Kotelchuck, "Safe Mothers, Healthy Babies," 116–20.

90. Michael K. Brown, *Race, Money and the American Welfare State* (Ithaca, NY: Cornell University Press, 1999), 17. See also Robert C. Lieberman, *Shifting the Color Line: Race and the American Welfare State* (Cambridge, MA: Harvard University Press, 1998).

91. Karen Davis and Cathy Shoen, *Health and the War on Poverty: A Ten-Year Appraisal* (Washington, DC: Brookings Institution, 1978), 160; Barbara Bergman, "How Two Countries Respond to Children's Needs," chap. 1 in *Saving Our Children from Poverty: What the United States Can Learn from France* (New York: Russell Sage Foundation, 1996), 1.

92. Rachel Garfield, Kendal Orgera, and Anthony Damico, "The Coverage Gap: Uninsured Poor Adults in States That Do Not Expand Medicaid," *Issue Brief* (Kaiser Family Foundation), January 14, 2020, https://www.kff.org/medicaid/issue-brief/the-coverage-gap-uninsured-poor-adults-in-states-that-do-not-expand-medicaid.

93. Madeline Guth, Rachel Garfield, and Robin Rudowitz, "The Effects of Medicaid Expansion under the ACA: Updated Findings from a Literature Review," *Issue Brief* (Kaiser Family Foundation), March 17, 2020, https://www.kff.org/medicaid/issue-brief/the-effects-of-medicaid-expansion-under-the-aca-updated-findings-from-a-literature-review-august-2019.

94. Chintin B. Bhatt and Consuelo M. Beck-Sagué, "Medicaid Expansion and Infant Mortality in the United States," *American Journal of Public Health* 108, no. 4 (April 2018): 565–67.

95. Julie L. Hudson and Asako S. Moriya, "Medicaid Expansion for Adults Had Measurable 'Welcome Mat' Effects on Their Children," *Health Affairs* 36, no. 9 (September 2017): 1643–51.

96. National Academies of Science, Engineering, and Medicine, *A Roadmap to Reducing Child Poverty* (Washington, DC: National Academies Press, 2019), 2–3.

97. Geoffrey Rose, "In Search of Health," chap. 8 in *The Strategy of Preventive Medicine* (New York: Oxford University Press, 1992).

98. Sardell, *U.S. Experiment in Social Medicine*, 36.

99. Norvez, *De la naissance à l'école*, 148–49.

2. Workers' Health in the United States and Germany

1. Ludwig Erhard, quoted in Alexander Rüstow, *Der mittelständische Unternehmer in der Sozialen Marktwirtschaft*, Aktionsgemeinschaft Soziale Marktwirtschaft (Ludwigsburg: Hoch, 1956): 51–61.

2. Clare Bambra, *Work, Worklessness, and the Political Economy of Health* (New York: Oxford University Press, 2011) 1, 9–11.

3. Sanders Marble, "Origins of the Physical Profile," *Military Medicine* 178, no. 8 (August 2013), 887–92; Michael R. Haines and Richard H. Steckel, "Childhood Mortality and

Nutritional Status as Indicators of Standard of Living: Evidence from World War I Recruits in the United States," NBER Historical Working Paper 121 (Cambridge, MA: National Bureau of Economic Research, 2000), 7–11.

4. Alexander Watson, *Enduring the Great War: Combat, Morale and Collapse in the German and British Armies, 1914–1918* (New York: Cambridge University Press, 2008).

5. National Research Council and Institute of Medicine, *U.S. Health in International Perspective: Shorter Lives, Poorer Health*, ed. Steven H. Woolf and Laudan Aron (Washington, DC: National Academies Press, 2013), 3; Cynthia Cox and Selena Gonzales, "The U.S. Has Highest Rate of Disease Burden among Comparable Countries, and the Gap Is Growing," Peterson-KFF Health System Tracker, July 7, 2015, http://www.healthsystem tracker.org/2015/07/the-u-s-has-highest-rate-of-disease-burden-among-comparable-countries-and-the-gap-is-growing; *Health in Germany—the Most Important Developments*, Federal Health Reporting (Berlin: Robert Koch Institute, 2015), https://www.rki.de/EN/Content/Health_ Monitoring/Health_Reporting/HealthInGermany/Health-in-Germany_most_important_ developments.pdf; "Germany," Institute of Health Metrics and Evaluation, http://www. healthdata.org/germany. When measuring the burden of disease on a population, epidemiologists employ a measure known as Disability Adjusted Life Years (DALYs). DALYs are a sum of lost healthy life years due to premature death plus the productive life years lost due to disabling health conditions. DALYs provide a more complete picture of a nation's health status than mortality rates because they show the burden of disease that arises from disabilities that may not ultimately cause death. For more on DALYs, see "Metrics: Disability Adjusted Life Year (DALY)," World Health Organization, http://www.who.int/healthinfo/global_burden_disease/metrics_daly/en.

6. This is not to say that heart disease did not previously exist. Indeed, whole body computed tomography (CT) scans of ancient mummies from three continents indicate the presence of atherosclerosis. It is just that infectious diseases, such as pneumonia and tuberculosis, overwhelmed heart disease as causes of death until the 1950s. The widespread use of the electrocardiogram in the twentieth century greatly improved the ability to diagnose acute myocardial infarction and thereby to recognize heart disease before death. See James Dalen, et al., "The Epidemic of the Twentieth Century: Coronary Heart Disease," *American Journal of Medicine* 127, no. 9 (September 2014): 807–12; Rachel Hajar, "Coronary Heart Disease: From Mummies to 21st Century," *Heart Views* 18, no. 2 (April–June 2017): 68–74.

7. "Labor Force Participation Rate, Total (% of Total Population Ages 15–64) (Modeled ILO Estimate)," 2019, World Bank, https://data.worldbank.org/indicator/SL.TLF.ACTI.ZS.

8. Marlene A. Lee and Mark Mather, "U.S. Labor Force Trends," *Population Bulletin* 63, no. 2 (June 2008); Mitra Toossi and Leslie Joyner, "Blacks in the Labor Force," *Spotlight on Statistics* (US Bureau of Labor Statistics), February 2018, https://www.bls.gov/spotlight/2018/ blacks-in-the-labor-force/pdf/blacks-in-the-labor-force.pdf; Marcus Casey and Bradley Hardy, "Reduced Unemployment Doesn't Equal Improved Well-Being for Black Americans," Brookings Institution, February 15, 2018, https://www.brookings.edu/blog/up-front/2018/02/15/ reduced-unemployment-doesnt-equal-improved-well-being-for-black-americans.

9. Aaron E. Cobet and Gregory A. Wilson, "Comparing 50 Years of Labor Productivity in U.S. and Foreign Manufacturing," *Monthly Labor Review*, June 2002, 51–65.

10. Darell M. West and Christian Lansang, "Global Manufacturing Scorecard: How the U.S. Compares to 18 Other Nations," *Brookings Institution Report*, July 10, 2018, https:// www.brookings.edu/research/global-manufacturing-scorecard-how-the-us-compares-to-18-other-nations.

11. Productivism is a theory according to which a constant increase in productivity is the primary goal of socioeconomic activity. *Lexico*, s.v. "productivism," https://en.oxforddictionaries. com/definition/productivism. See also Anthony Giddens, *Beyond Left and Right, the Future of Radical Politics* (Stanford, CA: Stanford University Press, 1994), 125–80.

12. Dietrich Milles, "Industrial Hygiene: A State Obligation? Industrial Pathology as a Problem in German Social Policy," in *State, Social Policy and Social Change in Germany, 1880–1994*, ed. W. R. Lee and Eve Rosenhaft (New York: Bergh, 1997), 165, 171–74.

13. Franz Koesch, *Was Weißtdu Du von Berufskrankheiten und Gewerbehygiene?* (Berlin: Arens, 1944), 3, quoted in ibid., 191.

14. Richard Hofstadter, *The Age of Reform: From Bryan to FDR* (New York: Knopf, 1955), 240.

15. Michael Stolleis, *Origins of the German Welfare State: Social Policy in Germany to 1945*, trans. Thomas Dunlap (Berlin: Springer, 2012), 82.

16. Ibid., 51.

17. Quoted in ibid., 52.

18. Ibid., 67.

19. Ibid., 53.

20. Max Hirsch, 1875, quoted in ibid., 61.

21. Bismarck's speech to the Reichstag, June 12, 1882, quoted in ibid., 62.

22. Industrialist Friedrich Wilhelm Harkort, quoted in ibid., 61.

23. Ferdinand Lassalle, quoted in ibid., 64.

24. Ibid., 67–71; Milles, "Industrial Hygiene," 166.

25. Stolleis, *Origins of the German Welfare State*, 67–68.

26. Allan Mitchell, *The Divided Path: The German Influence on Social Reform in France after 1870* (Chapel Hill: University of North Carolina Press, 1991); Paul V. Dutton, *Origins of the French Welfare State: The Struggle for Social Reform, 1914–1947* (New York: Cambridge University Press, 2002), 46–53.

27. Stolleis, *Origins of the German Welfare State*, 71–73.

28. Ibid., 74–75, 84.

29. Quoted in ibid., 64.

30. Ibid., 75.

31. Hofstadter, *Age of Reform*, 240.

32. Daniel T. Rogers, *Atlantic Crossings: Social Politics in a Progressive Age* (Cambridge, MA: Harvard University Press, 1998), 246.

33. Alonzo L. Hamby, "Progressivism: A Century of Change and Rebirth," in *Progressivism and the New Democracy*, ed. Sidney M. Milkis and Jerome M. Mileur (Amherst: University of Massachusetts Press, 1999), 41–80; Gary Gerstle, "The Protean Character of American Liberalism," *American Historical Review* 99, no. 4 (October 1994): 1043–73; Richard L. McCormick, "The Discovery That Business Corrupts Politics: A Reappraisal of the Origins of Progressivism," *American Historical Review* 86, no. 2 (April 1981): 247–74.

34. Walter G. Hoffmann, *Das Wachstum der deutschen Wirtschaft seit der Mitte des 19. Jahrhunderts* (Berlin: Springer, 1965), 173–74.

35. "Table 4: Population: 1790 to 1990," US Census Bureau, https://www.census.gov/population/censusdata/table-4.pdf.

36. Christopher C. Sellers, *Hazards of the Job: From Industrial Disease to Environmental Health Science* (Chapel Hill: University of North Carolina Press, 1997), 28.

37. Price V. Fishback and Shawn Everett Kantor, "The Adoption of Workers' Compensation in the United States, 1900–1930," NBER Working Paper 5840 (Cambridge, MA: National Bureau of Economic Research, 1996), 13, 16–18.

38. *The Works of Theodore Roosevelt, 1923–1926*, vol. 17, memorial ed. (New York: Scribner's Sons, 1970), 591.

39. Bryan Sawyers, "The Incovenient Worker—Can Mississippi's Public Policy Exceptions to the Employment-at-Will Doctrine Be Expanded to Encompass the Exercise of Workers' Compensation Rights?," *Mississippi Law Journal* 81, no. 6 (2012): 1563.

40. Rogers, *Atlantic Crossings*, 249–50.

41. Fishback and Kantor, "Adoption of Workers' Compensation in the United States," 11–24.

42. Beatrix Hoffman, *The Wages of Sickness: The Politics of Health Insurance in Progressive America* (Chapel Hill: University of North Carolina Press, 2001), 25.

43. Committee on Social Insurance, American Association for Labor Legislation, "Health Insurance: Tentative Draft of an Act," *American Labor Legislation Review*, June 1916, 241–42, 255–56, 248.

44. B. S. Warren and Edgar Sydenstriker, "Health Insurance, Its Relation to Public Health," *United States Public Health Service Bulletin*, no. 76 (March 1916): 49–50.

45. *Report of the Social Insurance Commission of the State of California, January 25, 1917* (Sacramento, CA: California State Printing Office, 1917), 122.

46. *Report of the Special Commission on Social Insurance, February 1917* (Boston: Wright and Potter Printing Co., State Printers, 1917), 23–24.

47. Paul Starr, *The Social Transformation of American Medicine* (New York: Basic Books, 1982), 253.

48. John Andrews quoted in Hoffman, *Wages of Sickness*, 178.

49. Gordon Craig, "Weltpolitik, Navalism, and the Coming of the War, 1897–1914," chap. 9 in *Germany, 1866–1945* (New York: Oxford University Press, 1980).

50. Robert N. Proctor, *The Nazi War on Cancer* (Princeton, NJ: Princeton University Press, 1991), 99.

51. Stolleis, *Origins of the German Welfare State*, 115–30.

52. 29 U.S.C. §§ 151–69 (1935).

53. Stolleis, *Origins of the German Welfare State*, 126–27.

54. *The Reich Constitution of August 11th 1919 (Weimar Constitution) with Modifications*, Articles 162 and 163, http://www.zum.de/psm/weimar/weimar_vve.php.

55. Stolleis, *Origins of the German Welfare State*, 141–42.

56. David Schoenbaum, "The Third Reich and Its Social Promises" and "The Third Reich and Labor," chaps. 1 and 3 in *Hitler's Social Revolution: Class and Status in Nazi Germany, 1933–1939* (New York: Norton, 1997); Richard Grunberger, *The 12-Year Reich: A Social History of Nazi Germany 1933–1945* (Boston: De Capo, 1995), 185–202.

57. Adam Tooze, "Recovery," pt. 1 in *The Wages of Destruction: The Making and Breaking of the Nazi Economy* (New York: Penguin, 2008).

58. Michael Burleigh, *The Third Reich: A New History* (New York: Hill and Wang, 2000), 218–25.

59. Proctor, *Nazi War on Cancer*, 105–6.

60. Martin Cherniack, *The Hawk's Nest Incident* (New Haven, CT: Yale University Press, 1986).

61. Proctor, *Nazi War on Cancer*, 8.

62. Ibid., 109–13.

63. Ibid., 118–19.

64. Manfred Schmidt, "Social Policy in the German Democratic Republic," in *The Rise and Fall of a Socialist Welfare State: The German Democratic Republic, 1949–1990, and German Unification, 1989–1994*, ed. Lutz Leisering, trans. David R. Antal and Ben Veghte (Berlin: Springer, 2013), 121, 73, 87–88, 63.

65. Ibid., 88.

66. Quoted in Hans Günter Hockerts, *Drei Wege deutscher Sozialstaatlichkei. NS-Diktatur, Bundesrepublik und DDR im Vergleich* (Munich: De Gruyter, 1998), 24.

67. I. Markovits quoted in Schmidt, "Social Policy in the German Democratic Republic," 63.

68. Ingo Haar and Michael Fahlbusch, *German Scholars and Ethnic Cleansing, 1920–1945* (New York: Berghahn, 2005), 10–12; Lutz Leisering, "Nation State and Social Policy:

An Ideational and Political History," in *Origins of the German Welfare State: Social Policy in Germany to 1945*, ed. Lutz Leisering, trans. Thomas Dunlap (Berlin: Springer, 2013), 2–8.

69. Hans F. Zacher, *Social Policy in the Federal Republic of Germany: The Constitution of the Social*, trans. Thomas Dunlap (Berlin: Springer-Verlag, 2013), 135.

70. Ibid., 124–27.

71. "Industrial Relations in Germany—Background Summary," European Trade Union Institute, April 4, 2019, https://www.etui.org/covid-social-impact/germany/industrial-relations-in-germany-background-summary-updated-april-2019.

72. Foreigners who travel in Germany often bemoan the widespread closure of stores on Sunday and their relatively restricted hours compared to elsewhere in Europe and the United States. In some cases, these restrictions stem from state and local regulations, but they also result from retail firms' works councils whose decisions both German consumers and retailers have grown accustomed to. Indeed, the leaders of Rossman and Hornbach, which are among the largest retail chains in Germany, would not expect substantially higher sales if their doors were flung open 24/7. "We are very happy with the current situation," Rossman told the German daily *Der Spiegel*. See "Why Are Shops in Germany Closed on Sundays?," *The Local.de*, October 17, 2017, https://www.thelocal.de/20171027/why-does-germany-have-such-strict-opening-hours-on-sundays.

73. Clare Bambra et al., "Tackling the Wider Social Determinants of Health and Health Inequalities: Evidence from Systematic Reviews," *Journal of Epidemiology and Community Health* 64, no. 4 (April 2010): 284–91.

74. *Journal of the American Medical Association* 99, no. 23 (December 1932): 1952.

75. Rogers, *Atlantic Crossings*, 429.

76. David Beito, *From Mutual Aid to the Welfare State: Fraternal Societies and Social Services, 1890–1967* (Chapel Hill: University of North Carolina Press, 2000), 219.

77. Franklin Delano Roosevelt, First Inaugural Address, Washington, DC, March 4, 1933.

78. Daniel S. Hirshfield, *The Lost Reform: The Campaign for Compulsory Health Insurance in the United States from 1932 to 1943* (Cambridge, MA: Harvard University Press, 1970), 44–49.

79. Jacob Hacker, *The Divided Welfare State: The Battle over Public and Private Social Benefits in the United States* (Cambridge, UK: Cambridge University Press, 2002), 209.

80. Jacob Hacker, "The Historical Logic of National Health Insurance: Structure and Sequence in the Development of British, Canadian, and U.S. Medical Policy," *Studies in American Political Development* 12, no. 2 (Spring 1998): 57–130, esp. 113.

81. Jill S. Quadagno, "Welfare Capitalism and the Social Security Act of 1935," *American Sociological Review* 49, no. 5 (October 1984): 632–47, esp. 641.

82. Colin Gordon, *Dead on Arrival: The Politics of Health Care in Twentieth-Century America* (Princeton, NJ: Princeton University Press, 2003), 185.

83. John Bound and Richard Burkhauser, "Chapter 51 Economic Analysis of Transfer Programs Targeted on People with Disabilities," in *Handbook of Labor Economics*, vol. 3 (Amsterdam: Elsevier, 1999), 3453–64.

84. C. W. Crownhart, "The Relation of Compensation to Safety," *National Safety Council Proceedings* 3 (1914), 293–96; and Magnus Alexander, "The Economic Value of Industrial Safety," *National Safety Council Proceedings* 1 (1912), 204–11, both quoted in Mark Aldrich, *Safety First: Technology, Labor, and Business in the Building of American Work Safety, 1870–1939* (Baltimore: Johns Hopkins University Press, 1997), 104.

85. Aldrich, *Safety First*, 122.

86. Aldrich, *Safety First*, 164–66.

87. "Special Meeting of the Safety Committee," May 19, 1931, box 103, Bancroft Papers, Hagley Museum and Library, quoted in Aldrich, *Safety First*, 130.

88. Letter from E. E. Evans, director, Medical Division, Chamber Works, on behalf of W. C. Brothers, manager of Chamber Works, to A. Mangelsdorff, June 18, 1947, quoted in David Michaels, *Doubt Is Their Product: How Industry's Assault on Science Threatens Your Health* (New York: Oxford University Press, 2008), 19–20.

89. Michaels, *Doubt Is Their Product*, 14–19; Proctor, *Nazi War on Cancer*, 109–13.

90. *Reflections on OSHA's History*, OSHA 3360 (US Department of Labor, Occupational Safety and Health Administration, 2009), 14, https://www.osha.gov/history/OSHA_HISTORY_3360s.pdf.

91. *Marshall v. Barlow's Inc.*, 436 U.S. 307 (1978), syllabus, p. 236, U.S. 308; Morton Mintz, "Supreme Court Says a Warrant Is Needed for OSHA Inspection," *Washington Post*, May 24, 1978.

92. International Labour Organisation, *Introductory Report: Decent Work—Safe Work* (Geneva: ILO, 2005), 33–35.

93. Daniel Schneider and Kristen Harknett, "Consequences of Routine Work-Schedule Instability for Worker Health and Well-Being," *American Sociological Review* 84, no. 1 (February 2019): 82–114; Lars Alfredsson et al., "Types of Occupation and Near-Future Hospitalization for Myocardial Infarction and Some Other Diagnoses," *International Journal of Epidemiology* 14, no. 3 (September 1985): 378–88; M. Haan, "Job Strain and Cardiovascular Disease: A 10-year Prospective Study," paper presented at the Eighteenth Annual Meeting of the Society for Epidemiologic Research, 1985, Chapel Hill, North Carolina; Robert A. Karasek, "Job Demands, Job Decision Latitude, and Mental Strain: Implications for Job Redesign," *Administrative Science Quarterly* 24, no. 2 (June 1979): 285–306; Robert A. Karasek, "Control in the Workplace and Its Health-related Aspects," in *Job Control and Worker Health*, ed. Steven L. Sauter et al. (Hoboken, NJ: Wiley, 1989), 129–59; Robert Karasek and Töres Theorell, *Healthy Work* (New York: Basic Books, 1989); Andrea Z. La Croix and Suzanne G. Haynes, "Occupational Exposure to High Demand/Low Control Work and Coronary Heart Disease Incidence in the Framingham Cohort," paper presented at the Eighteenth Annual Meeting of the Society for Epidemiologic Research, Houston, 1984; Rudy Fenwick and Mark Tausig, "The Macroeconomic Context of Job Stress," *Journal of Health and Social Behavior* 35 (1994): 266–82.

94. Sebastian Maiss and Stefan Röhrborn, "Germany: New Legislation Adjusts Temporary Employment and Contracts for Work and Labour," *Insights* (newsletter of the Littler Mendelson law firm), 2018, 1–2.

95. *Contingent Workforce: Size, Characteristics, Earnings and Benefits* (Washington, DC: US Government Accountability Office, 2015), 15, https://www.gao.gov/assets/670/669766.pdf.

96. Rudy Fenwick and Mark Tausig, "Scheduling Stress: Family and Health Outcomes of Shift Work and Schedule Control," *American Behavioral Scientist* 44, no. 7 (March 2001): 1179–98; Marilyn Fox, Deborah Dwyer, and Daniel Ganster, "Effects of Stressful Job Demands and Control on Physiological and Attitudinal Outcomes in a Hospital Setting," *Academy Management Journal* 36, no. 2 (April 1993): 289–318.

97. Bert Schreurs et al., "Job Insecurity and Employee Health: The Buffering Potential of Job Control and Job Self-Efficacy," *Work and Stress* 24, no. 1 (January–March 2010): 56–72; Jana Mäcken, "Work Stress among Older Employees in Germany: Effects on Health and Retirement Age," *PLOS One* 14, no. 2 (2019): e0211487, https://journals.plos.org/plosone/article/file?id=10.1371/journal.pone.0211487&type=printable.

98. Joel Rogers and Wolfgang Streeck, *Works Councils: Consultation, Representation, and Cooperation in Industrial Relations* (Chicago: University of Chicago Press, 1995), 4. Emphasis in original.

99. Martin Behrens, "Still Married after All These Years? Union Organizing and the Role of Works Councils in German Industrial Relations," *Industrial and Labor Relations Review* 62, no. 3 (April 2009): 275–93.

3. After Work in the United States and Sweden

1. Healthy AgeWatch Index 2015, http://www.helpage.org/global-agewatch.

2. Robin Osborn et al., "Older Americans Were Sicker and Faced More Financial Barriers to Health Care than Counterparts in Other Countries," *Health Affairs* 36, no. 12 (December 2017): 2123–32. The study included Australia, Canada, France, Germany, the Netherlands, New Zealand, Norway, Sweden, Switzerland, the United Kingdom, and the United States.

3. Ibid., 2128–29.

4. Paula Braverman and Laura Gottlieb, "The Social Determinants of Health: It's Time to Consider the Causes of the Causes," *Public Health Report* 129, supplement 2 (January–February 2014): 19–31; Thomas Lehnert et al., "Review: Health Care Utilization and Costs of Elderly Persons with Multiple Chronic Conditions," *Medical Care Research and Review* 68, no. 4 (August 2011): 387–420; Elizabeth Bradley and Lauren Taylor, *The American Health Care Paradox: Why Spending More Is Getting Us Less* (New York: Public Affairs, 2015); Steven H. Woolf et al., *How Are Income and Wealth Linked to Health and Longevity*, Income and Health Initiative, Brief 1 (Urban Institute and Center on Society and Health, Virginia Commonwealth University, 2015), https://www.urban.org/sites/default/files/publication/49116/2000178-How-are-Income-and-Wealth-Linked-to-Health-and-Longevity.pdf.

5. Craig M. Hales, Margaret D. Carroll, Cheryl D. Fryar, and Cynthia L. Ogden, *Prevalence of Obesity among Adults and Youth: United States, 2015–2016*, NCHS Data Brief 288 (Hyattsville, MD: US Department of Health and Human Services, Centers for Disease Control and Prevention, National Center for Health Statistics, October 2017). Obesity is defined as body mass index of 30 or greater.

6. "Overweight and Obesity," Folkhälsomyndigheten (Public Health Agency of Sweden), May 2018, https://www.folkhalsomyndigheten.se/the-public-health-agency-of-sweden/living-conditions-and-lifestyle/obesity.

7. Axel Börsch-Supan et al., *First Results from the Survey of Health, Ageing and Retirement in Europe (2004–2007): Starting the Longitudinal Dimension* (Mannheim: Mannheim Research Institute for the Economics of Aging, 2008), 27, http://www.share-project.org/uploads/tx_sharepublications/BuchSHAREganz250808.pdf; Suzanne R. Kunkel et al., *Aging, Society, and the Life Course* (Berlin: Springer, 2015), 1; "Proposed Definition of an Elderly Person in Africa for the MDS Project," World Health Organization, https://www.who.int/healthinfo/survey/ageingdefnolder/en; Hajimi Orimo et al., "Reviewing the Definition of 'Elderly'," *Geriatrics and Gerontology International* 6, no. 3 (August 2006): 149–58.

8. 2017 Profile of Older Americans (U.S. Department of Health and Human Services, Administration for Community Living, 2018), 1, https://acl.gov/sites/default/files/Aging%20and%20Disability%20in%20America/2017OlderAmericansProfile.pdf; "Sweden Age Structure," in Sweden Population, CountryMeters.info, https://countrymeters.info/en/Sweden#age_structure.

9. *World Report on Ageing and Health* (Geneva: World Health Organization, 2015), https://www.who.int/ageing/events/world-report-2015-launch/en.

10. David S. Landes, *The Unbound Prometheus: Technical Change and Industrial Development in Western Europe from 1750 to the Present* (New York: Cambridge University Press, 2003).

11. These developments are wonderfully described by E. P. Thompson, "Time, Work-Discipline, and Industrial Capitalism," *Past and Present* 38 (December 1967) 56–97.

12. William Graebner, *A History of Retirement: The Meaning and Function of an American Institution, 1885–1978* (New Haven, CT: Yale University Press, 1980); Dora L. Costa, *The Evolution of Retirement: An American Economic History, 1880–1990* (Chicago: University of Chicago Press, 1998).

13. Peter Laslett, "The Emergence of the Third Age," *Aging and Society* 7 (1987), 133–60; Anne-Marie Guillemard, *Le déclin du social, formation et crise des politiques de la vieillesse* (Paris: Presses universitaires de France, 1986), 191.

14. James O'Connell, "The Manhood Tribute to the Modern Machine: Influences Determining the Length of Trade Life Among Machinists," *Annals of the American Academy of Political and Social Science* 27 (May 2006): 29–33.

15. Carole Haber, "Mandatory Retirement in Nineteenth-Century America: The Conceptual Basis for a New Work Cycle," *Journal of Social History* 12, no. 1 (October 1978): 77–96, esp. 79.

16. Roger L. Ransom and Richard Sutch, "The Impact of Aging on the Employment of Men in American Working-Class Communities at the End of the Nineteenth Century," in *Aging in the Past: Demography, Society, and Old Age*, ed. David I. Kertzer and Peter Laslett (Berkeley: University of California Press, 1995), 304–16.

17. "First National Bank of Chicago Pension Fund (1899)," *Twenty-Third Annual Report of the Commissioner of Labor*, 645–46, as cited by Haber, "Mandatory Retirement in Nineteenth-Century America," 83; Haber, "Mandatory Retirement in Nineteenth-Century America," 82.

18. Teresa Ghilarducci, *Labor's Capital: The Economics and Politics of Private Pensions* (Cambridge, MA: MIT Press, 1992), 15.

19. "Western Electric Company Pension System (1906)," *Twenty-Third Annual Report of the Commissioner of Labor*, 646–47, quoted in Haber, "Mandatory Retirement in Nineteenth-Century America," 82–83.

20. Quoted in Haber, "Mandatory Retirement in Nineteenth-Century America," 83.

21. Jennifer Klein, *For All These Rights: Business, Labor, and the Shaping of America's Public-Private Welfare State* (Princeton, NJ: Princeton University Press, 2003), 54–55, 120–21; Ghilarducci, *Labor's Capital*, 30–31.

22. Massachusetts Commission on Old Age Pensions, Annuities, and Insurance, *Report of the Commission on Old Age Pensions, Annuities, and Insurance* (Boston: Wright and Potter Printing Co., State Printers, 1910), 270–71, cited by Haber, "Mandatory Retirement in Nineteenth-Century America," 88.

23. Lewis Meriam, *Principles Governing the Retirement of Public Employees* (New York: Appleton, 1918), 385, xii.

24. Tamara K. Hareven and Peter Uhlenberg, "Transition to Widowhood and Family Support Systems in Twentieth Century, Northeastern United States," in Kertzer and Laslett, *Aging in the Past*, 273–91.

25. Roy Lubove, *The Struggle for Social Security, 1900–1935* (Pittsburgh: University of Pittsburgh Press, 1986), 118–20.

26. George Alter, "Trends in Old Age Mortality in the United States, 1900–1935: Evidence from Railroad Pensions," in Kertzer and Laslett, *Aging in the Past*, 332.

27. Costa, *Evolution of Retirement*, 16–17.

28. Edwin Amenta, *When Movements Matter: The Townsend Plan and the Rise of Social Security* (Princeton, NJ: Princeton University Press, 2006), 36–45.

29. "Payroll Tax Rates: 1937 to 2019," Tax Policy Center, Urban Institute and Brookings Institution, https://www.taxpolicycenter.org/statistics/payroll-tax-rates.

30. "Policy Basics: Top Ten Facts about Social Security," Center on Budget and Policy Priorities, https://www.cbpp.org/research/social-security/policy-basics-top-ten-facts-about-social-security.

31. Jill S. Quadagno, "Welfare Capitalism and the Social Security Act of 1935," *American Sociological Review* 49, no. 5 (October 1984): 632–47, esp. 634–36.

32. Colin Gordon, *Dead on Arrival: The Politics of Health Care in Twentieth-Century America* (Princeton, NJ: Princeton University Press, 2003), 185.

33. Klein, *For All These Rights,* 103–5.

34. Andreas Bergh, "What Are the Policy Lessons from Sweden? On the Rise, Fall and Revival of a Capitalist Welfare State," *New Political Economy* 19, no. 5 (2014): 662–94.

35. Johannes Hagen, "A History of the Swedish Pension System," Working Paper 2013:7 (Uppsala: Uppsala Center for Fiscal Studies, Department of Economics, 2013), 15–16, http://uu.diva-portal.org/smash/get/diva2:621560/FULLTEXT01.pdf.

36. Per Gunnar Edebalk, "Emergence of a Welfare State—Social Insurance in Sweden in the 1910s," *Journal of Social Policy* 29, no. 4 (November 2000): 537–51.

37. Ibid.

38. Peter Baldwin, *The Politics of Social Solidarity: Class Bases of the European Welfare State, 1875–1975* (New York: Cambridge University Press, 1990); Sven E. O. Hort, *Social Policy, Welfare State, and Civil Society in Sweden,* vol. 1, *History, Policies and Institutions, 1884–1988* (Lund, Sweden: Arkiv Academic Press, 2014), 41–45.

39. Hort, *Social Policy, Welfare State, and Civil Society in Sweden,* vol. 1, 80–81.

40. Ibid., 125.

41. Hagen, "History of the Swedish Pension System," 31.

42. Hort, *Social Policy, Welfare State, and Civil Society in Sweden,* vol. 1, 104–5.

43. Hagen, "History of the Swedish Pension System," 38–54.

44. Hort, *Social Policy, Welfare State, and Civil Society in Sweden,* vol. 1, 111–12; Anders Anell, Anna H. Glenngård, and Sherry Merkur, *Sweden: Health System Review,* Health Systems in Transition 14, no. 5 (Copenhagen: World Health Organization on behalf of the European Observatory on Health Systems and Policies, 2012), http://www.euro.who.int/__data/assets/pdf_file/0008/164096/e96455.pdf.

45. Anne R. Somers and Herman M. Somers, "Health Insurance: Are Cost and Quality Controls Necessary?," *Industrial and Labor Relations Review* 13, no. 4 (July 1960): 581.

46. Jacob Hacker, *The Divided Welfare State: The Battle over Public and Private Social Benefits in the United States* (New York: Cambridge University Press, 2002), 245.

47. Sylvester J. Schieber, *The Predictable Surprise: The Unraveling of the U.S. Retirement System* (New York: Oxford University Press, 2012), 301.

48. "Health Areas for Discussion," September 22, 1965, box 120:3, Wilbur Cohen Papers, State Historical Society of Wisconsin, Madison, quoted in Colin Gordon, *Dead on Arrival,* 239.

49. "Lyndon B. Johnson Tapes," Social Security Administration Special Collections, 7 WH6503.14, March 29, 1965, https://www.ssa.gov/history/LBJ/lbj.html.

50. "Statement of the American Medical Association: Re: H.R. 4222, 87th Congress Medical Aid for the Aged to be Financed Through Social Security," *Journal of the American Medical Association* 177, no. 6 (August 12, 1961): 368–69; *House Committee on Ways and Means, Health Services for the Aged Under the Social Security Insurance System,* 87th Cong. (1961) (statement of R. B. Robbins), vols. 3–4, 2219–20.

51. Gordon, *Dead on Arrival,* 235.

52. Quoted in Robert Dallek, *Flawed Giant: Lyndon Johnson and His Times* (New York: Oxford University Press, 1998), 209–10.

53. Theodore Marmor, "The Politics of Legislative Certainty," chap. 4 in *The Politics of Medicare* (New York: Aldine Transaction, 2000).

54. Wilbur Cohen, "Random Reflections on the Great Society's Politics and Health Programs after Twenty Years," in *The Great Society and Its Legacy: Twenty Years of U.S. Social Policy,* ed. Marshal Kaplan and Peggy Cuciti (Durham, NC: Duke University Press, 1986); Robert Cunningham III and Robert Cunningham Jr., *The Blues: A History of the Blue Cross*

and Blue Shield System (De Kalb: Northern Illinois Press, 1997), 151; Paul Starr, *The Social Transformation of American Medicine* (New York: Basic Books, 1982), 375.

55. Marmor, "The Politics of Legislative Certainty," 110–13.

56. Robin A. Cohen et al., "Health Insurance Coverage Trends, 1959–2007: Estimates from the National Health Interview Survey," *National Health Statistics Reports*, no. 17 (July 1, 2009): 4, https://www.cdc.gov/nchs/data/nhsr/nhsr017.pdf.

57. "An Overview of Medicare," *Issue Brief* (Kaiser Family Foundation), February 2019, https://www.kff.org/medicare/issue-brief/an-overview-of-medicare.

58. Ibid.

59. Invoice, Medicare Plan F, California Blue Shield, October 2019.

60. "Medicare Spend-Down in New York State," flier, Medicaid Rights Center, 2020, http://www.medicarerights.org/fliers/Medicaid/Medicaid-Spend-Down-(NY).pdf.

61. Gretchen Davidson et al., "A Dozen Facts about Medicare Advantage," Data Note (Kaiser Family Foundation), November 2018, https://www.kff.org/medicare/issue-brief/a-dozen-facts-about-medicare-advantage.

62. "What Is Long-Term Care?," National Institute on Aging, 2019, https://www.nia.nih.gov/health/what-long-term-care.

63. "Long-term Care," US Centers for Medicare and Medicaid Services, https://www.medicare.gov/coverage/long-term-care; Medicare and Home Health Care (Baltimore: US Centers for Medicare and Medicaid Services, 2019), 5–12, https://www.medicare.gov/Pubs/pdf/10969-Medicare-and-Home-Health-Care.pdf.

64. Wendy Fox-Grage and Kathleen Ujvari, "Older Americans Act," *Insight on the Issues* (AARP Public Policy Institute) 92 (May 2014), https://www.aarp.org/content/dam/aarp/research/public_policy_institute/health/2014/the-older-americans-act-AARP-ppi-health.pdf.

65. Jeffrey R. Brown and Amy Finkelstein, "Why Is the Market for Long-Term Care Insurance So Small?," *Journal of Public Economics* 91, no. 10 (November 2007): 1967–91.

66. "Medicaid's Role in Nursing Care," Kaiser Family Foundation, June 20, 2017, https://www.kff.org/infographic/medicaids-role-in-nursing-home-care.

67. Dennis Shea et al., "Exploring Assistance in Sweden and the United States," *Gerontologist* 43, no. 5 (October 2003): 712–21.

68. Adam Davey et al., "Aging in Sweden: Local Variation, Local Control," *Gerontologist* 54, no. 4 (October 2013): 525–32.

69. Ibid.; Jyoti Savla, et al., "Home Health Services in Sweden: Responsiveness to Changing Demographics and Needs," *European Journal of Ageing* 5, no. 1 (March 2008): 47–55; "Elderly Care in Sweden," 2019, https://sweden.se/society/elderly-care-in-sweden.

70. Ichiro Kawichi et al., "Social Capital, Income Inequality, and Mortality, *American Journal of Public Health* 87, no. 9 (September 1997): 1491–98; Robert Putnam, *Bowling Alone: The Collapse and Revival of American Community* (New York: Simon & Schuster, 2000); Jennie Popay, "Social Capital: The Role of Narrative and Historical Research," *Journal of Epidemiology and Community Health* 54, no. 6 (June 2000): 401; T. A. Glass et al., "Social Engagement and Depressive Symptoms in Late Life: Longitudinal Findings," *Journal of Ageing and Health* 18, no. 4 (August 2006): 604–28; E. A. Miller and W. G. Weissert, "Predicting Elderly People's Risk for Nursing Home Placement, Hospitalization, Functional Impairment, and Mortality: a Synthesis," *Medical Care Research and Review* 57, no. 3 (September 2000): 259–97.

71. Ichiro Kawichi and Lisa Berkman, *Social Cohesion, Social Capital, and Health* (New York: Oxford University Press, 2000).

72. Maria Felice Arrezo and Cristina Giudici, "Social Capital and Perceived Health among European Older Adults," *Social Indicators Research* 130, no. 2 (January 2017): 665–85.

73. Olivia Dean, Claire Noel-Miller, and Keith Lind, "Who Relies on Medicare? A Profile of the Medicare Population," fact sheet, AARP Policy Institute, November 2017, https://www.aarp.org/content/dam/aarp/ppi/2017/11/who-relies-on-medicare-a-profile-of-the-medicare-population.pdf.

74. Shea et al., "Exploring Assistance in Sweden and the United States," 713.

75. Hui-Xin Wang et al., "Late-Life Engagement in Social and Leisure Activities Is Associated with a Decreased Risk of Dementia: A Longitudinal Study from the Kungsholmen Project," *American Journal of Epidemiology* 155, no. 12 (June 2002): 1081–87; Morten Wahrendorf, "Who in Europe Works beyond the State Pension Age and under Which Conditions: Results from SHARE," *Population Ageing* 10, no. 3 (September 2016), 269–85.

76. Karsten Hank and Marcel Erlinghagen, "Volunteer Work," in Börsch-Supan et al., *First Results from the Survey of Health, Ageing and Retirement in Europe*, 259–64. Surveys that query volunteering among Americans measure annual participation, whereas European surveys query monthly participation. The resulting data are incomparable.

77. Annika Edström and Madelene Gustafsson, "Elderly Living in Sweden: Present Solutions and Future Trends," MS thesis, KTH Royal Institute of Technology, Stockholm, 39.

78. Cecilia Henning et al., "Senior Housing in Sweden: A New Concept for Aging in Place," *Social Work in Public Health* 24, no. 3 (March 2009): 235–54.

79. Andrew E. Scharlach and Amanda J. Lehning, "Ageing-Friendly Communities and Social Inclusion in the United States of America," *Ageing and Society* 33, no. 1 (January 2013): 110–36.

80. Ibid., 130–31.

81. Gary Mormino, "Sunbelt Dreams and Altered States: A Social and Cultural History of Florida, 1950–2000," *Florida Historical Quarterly* 81, no. 1 (Summer 2002): 3–21. See also Gary Mormino, *Land of Sunshine, State of Dreams: A Social History of Modern Florida* (Gainesville: University Press of Florida, 2008).

82. John M. Findlay, *Magic Lands: Western Cityscapes and American Culture after 1940* (Berkeley: University of California Press, 1992), 10, 166–68.

83. Paul V. Dutton, "*Des sanatoriums à Sun City: L'invention de la 'retraite active' en Arizona*," *Le Mouvement Social* 258, no. 1 (January–March 2017): 85–107.

84. Quoted in Doris Paine, "The Sun City Story," supplement, *Phoenix Magazine*, 1978, S-4.

85. Jennie Keith-Ross, *Old People, New Lives: Community Creation in a Retirement Residence* (Chicago: University of Chicago Press, 1977), 198.

86. Judith Ann Trolander, "Age 55 or Better: Active Adult Communities and City Planning," *Journal of Urban History* 37, no. 6 (November 2011): 952–74, esp. 964.

87. "Quick Facts, Maricopa County, Arizona," US Census Bureau, [2019], https://www.census.gov/quickfacts/fact/table/maricopacountyarizona,US/RHI725218.

88. The website 55places.com provides potential buyers with an overview of each of these, http://www.55places.com/arizona. See also Trolander, "Age 55 or Better."

89. Edström and Gustafsson, "Elderly Living in Sweden," 29.

90. Scharlach and Lehning, "Ageing-Friendly Communities," 130.

91. Dominique Anxo and Harald Niklasson, "The Swedish Model: Revival after the Turbulent 1990s?," Discussion Paper Series, International Institute for Labor Studies of the International Labor Organization, Geneva, 2008, 3–4; Stefan Fölster and Johan Kreicbergs, *Twenty Five Years of Swedish Reforms* (Stockholm: Reforminstitute, 2014), 1, https://www.reforminstitutet.se/wp/wp-content/uploads/2014/03/Twentyfiveyearsofreform140301.pdf.

92. Hagen, "History of the Swedish Pension System," 52–54.

93. Anxo and Niklasson, "Swedish Model," vi.

94. Ibid., 14–16.

95. Gunn-Britt Trydegård, "Swedish Care Reforms in the 1990s: A First Evaluation of Their Consequences for Elderly People," *Revue française des affaires sociales* 57, no. 4 (2003/4): 443–60.

96. Davey et al., "Aging in Sweden."

97. Fölster and Kreicbergs, *Twenty Five Years of Swedish Reforms*, 4–10.

98. Richard Heller, "The New Face of Swedish Socialism," *Forbes*, March 19, 2001, https://www.forbes.com/global/%202001/0319/034.html.

99. Göran Normann and Daniel J. Mitchell, "Pension Reform in Sweden: Lessons for American Policymakers," *Heritage Foundation Backgrounder: Executive Summary*, no. 1381 (June 29, 2000).

100. Tetsuji Yamada et al., "Access Disparity and Health Inequality of the Elderly: Unmet Needs and Delayed Healthcare," *International Journal of Environmental Research and Public Health* 12, no. 2 (February 2015): 1745–72.

101. Schieber, *Predictable Surprise*, 15.

102. Schieber, "And Then, a Predictable Defined Benefit Surprise," chap. 19 in *Predictable Surprise*.

103. Ibid., 205.

104. "The Time Bomb inside Public Pension Plans," August 23, 2018, *Knowledge@Wharton*, University of Pennsylvania, 2019, http://knowledge.wharton.upenn.edu/article/the-time-bomb-inside-public-pension-plans.

105. Schieber, "Public Pensions: The Good, the Bad, and the Ugly," chap. 20 in *Predictable Surprise*.

106. "1 in 3 Americans Have Less Than $5,000 in Retirement Savings," Northwestern Mutual, May 8, 2018, news release, https://news.northwesternmutual.com/2018-05-08-1-In-3-Americans-Have-Less-Than-5-000-In-Retirement-Savings.

107. Stephen C. Goss, "The 2018 Annual Report of the Board of Trustees of the Federal Old-Age and Survivors Insurance and Federal Disability Trust Funds," *Social Security Bulletin*, 70, no. 3 (2010), https://www.ssa.gov/policy/docs/ssb/v70n3/v70n3p111.html.

108. Bernt Lundgren, "The Making of National Health Policy: Experiences from the Swedish Determinants-Based Public Health Policy," *International Journal of Health Services* 39, no. 3 (2009): 491–507.

Conclusion

1. Anne Case and Angus Deaton, "Rising Morbidity and Mortality in Midlife among White Non-Hispanic Americans in the 21st Century," *Proceedings of the National Academy of Sciences* 112, no. 49 (September 2015): 15078–83.

2. "Health," OECD Better Life Index, http://www.oecdbetterlifeindex.org/topics/health.

3. Steven H. Woolf et al., How Are Income and Wealth Linked to Health and Longevity, Income and Health Initiative, Brief 1 (Urban Institute and Center on Society and Health, 2015), https://www.urban.org/sites/default/files/publication/49116/2000178-How-are-Income-and-Wealth-Linked-to-Health-and-Longevity.pdf.

4. Julia B. Isaacs, "International Comparisons of Economic Mobility," in *Getting Ahead or Losing Ground: Economic Mobility in America*, by Julia B. Isaacs, Isabel V. Sawhill, and Ron Haskins (Washington, DC: Brookings Institution Press, 2008), 37–46, https://www.brookings.edu/wp-content/uploads/2016/06/02_economic_mobility_sawhill.pdf.

5. Ibid.; Thomas Piketty, Emmanuel Saez, and Gabriel Zucman, "Distributional National Accounts: Methods and Estimates for the United States," *Quarterly Journal of Economics* 133, no. 2 (May 2018) 553–609; "Does America Promote Mobility as Well as Other

Nations," Pew Charitable Trusts, Economic Mobility Project, November 2011, https://www.pewtrusts.org/~/media/legacy/uploadedfiles/pcs_assets/2011/critafinal1pdf.pdf.

6. Anthony B. Atkinson et al., "Top Incomes in the Long Run of History," *Journal of Economics Literature* 49, no. 1 (2011): 3–71, esp. 9.

7. "Advancing Health in America: Addressing Social Determinants of Health," American Hospital Association, 2018, https://www.aha.org/addressing-social-determinants-health-presentation; "What Montefiore's 300% ROI from Social Determinants Investments Means for the Future of Other Hospitals," *Health Care Finance News*, July 5, 2018; "How Addressing Social Determinants of Health Cuts Health Care Costs," Revcycle Intelligence-Xtelligent Healthcare Media, June 25, 2018, https://revcycleintelligence.com/news/how-addressing-social-determinants-of-health-cuts-healthcare-costs.

8. "About Social Determinants of Health," World Health Organization, https://www.who.int/social_determinants/sdh_definition/en; Brian Castrucci and John Auerbach, "Meeting Individual Social Needs Falls Short of Addressing Social Determinants of Health," *Health Affairs Blog*, January 16, 2019, https://www.healthaffairs.org/do/10.1377/hblog20190115.234942/full.

9. Len M. Nichols and Lauren A. Taylor, "Social Determinants as Public Goods: A New Approach to Financing Key Investments in Health Communities," *Health Affairs* 37, no. 8 (August 2018): 1223–30.

10. Rebecca Masters et al., "Return on Investment of Public Health Interventions: A Systematic Review," *Journal of Epidemiology and Community Health* 71, no. 8 (August 2017); 827–34; Paula Braveman and Laura Gottlieb, "It's Time to Consider the Causes of the Causes," *Public Health Report*, 129, supplement 2, (January–February 2014): 19–31.

11. Ilona Kickbusch and Kevin Buckett, *Implementing Health in All Policies, Adelaide 2010* (Adelaide: Department of Health, Government of South Australia, 2010), 14, https://www.who.int/sdhconference/resources/implementinghiapadel-sahealth-100622.pdf.

12. Vicente Navarro, "What We Mean by Social Determinants of Health," *International Journal of Health Services* 39, no. 3 (March 2009), 423–41.

13. Castrucci and Auerbach, "Meeting Individual Social Needs Falls Short."

14. Kimmo Leppo et al., eds., *Health in All Policies*, Ministry of Social Affairs and Health, Finland, 2013, http://www.euro.who.int/__data/assets/pdf_file/0007/188809/Health-in-All-Policies-final.pdf.

15. "Health in All Policies: Framework for Country Action," World Health Organization, May 9, 2013), 2, http://www.who.int/healthpromotion/conferences/8gchp/130509_hiap_framework_for_country_action_draft.pdf; Institute of Medicine, *Improving Health in the United States: The Role of Health Impact Assessment* (Washington, DC: National Academies Press, 2011).

16. "Budget 2019," Treasury (New Zealand), https://treasury.govt.nz/publications/budgets/budget-2019; "Adelaide Recommendations on Healthy Public Policy," World Health Organization, 1988, http://www.who.int/healthpromotion/conferences/previous/adelaide/en/index3.html.

17. John Kemm et al., eds., *Health Impact Assessment: Concepts, Theory, Techniques, and Applications* (New York: Oxford University Press, 2004).

18. R. Quigley et al., *Health Impact Assessment: International Best Practice Principles*, Special Series 5 (Fargo, ND: International Association for Impact Assessment, 2006).

19. Janet Collins and Jeffrey Koplan, "Health Impact Assessment: A Step toward Health in All Policies," *Journal of the American Medical Association* 302, no. 3 (July 15, 2009): 315–17.

20. "Health in All Policies Task Force," State of California Department of Justice, Office of the Attorney General, https://oag.ca.gov/environment/communities/policies.

21. For a helpful distinction between condition and problem that can spur state action, see John Kingdon, *Agendas, Alternatives, and Public Policies* (Boston: Addison Wesley, 1995).

22. David Pinkney, *Napoleon III and the Rebuilding of Paris* (Princeton, NJ: Princeton University Press, 1958).

23. Richard Evans, *Death in Hamburg: Society and Politics in the Cholera Years, 1830–1910* (New York: Penguin, 2005).

24. Elmer A. Beck, *The Sewer Socialists: A History of the Socialist Party of Wisconsin, 1897–1940* (Fennimore, WI: Westburg Associates, 1982).

25. Ilona Kickbusch, "Health in All Policies, the Evolution of the Concept of Horizontal Governance," in Kickbusch and Buckett, *Implementing Health in All Policies, Adelaide 2010*, 11–24.

26. Göran Normann and Daniel J. Mitchell, "Pension Reform in Sweden: Lessons for American Policymakers," *Heritage Foundation Backgrounder: Executive Summary*, no. 1381 (June 29, 2000).

27. Thomas Piketty, *Capital in the Twenty-First Century* (Cambridge, MA: Harvard University Press, 2017), Kindle ed., 630.

28. Sherry Xin Li et al., "Who's in Charge? Donor Targeting Enhances Voluntary Giving to Government," *SSRN Electronic Journal*, March 29, 2013, http://dx.doi.org/10.2139/ssrn.2293407; Cait Lamberton et al., "Eliciting Taxpayer Preferences Increases Taxpayer Compliance," Harvard Business School, Working Paper 14–106, April 23, 2014; "What Is the Tax Gap?," Tax Policy Center, Urban Institute and Brookings Institution, https://www.taxpolicycenter.org/briefing-book/what-tax-gap.

29. Glen P. Mays et al., "Preventable Death Rates Fell Where Communities Expanded Population Health Activities through Multisector Networks," *Health Affairs* 35, no.11 (November 2016): 2005–13.

30. "Healthy People 2030 Framework," US Department of Health and Human Services, Office of Disease Prevention and Health Promotion, https://www.healthypeople.gov/2020/About-Healthy-People/Development-Healthy-People-2030/Framework.

31. Mariana Mazzucato, *The Entrepreneurial State* (New York: Public Affairs, 2015), 15.

INDEX

Page numbers in *italics* indicate illustrative material.

Ratcliff, Kathryn Strother, 7
Reagan, Ronald, 127, 129
Reconstruction Finance Corporation, 96
Rerum Novarum (papal encyclical, 1891), 43
resource curse, 121
retirement and health in Germany:
  age of retirement, 78, 110; chronic disease rates, 109; in East versus West Germany, 92; Nazis, treatment of elders under, 90–91; pensions as part of social insurance programs, 77–78, 82, 115; US retirement arrangements and, 117, 119; worker health and, 109
retirement and health in US and Sweden, 24, 26, 107–45, 147; age-restricted communities, 135–38; aging in place, 107, 132, 134–35, 137; aging trends in Europe versus US, 4–5; childhood/working years health care affecting, 108–10; chronic disease rates, 109–10; defining "elderly" and "old age," 110–11; employer pension plans, 114–15; financial security in old age in Sweden (1870–1950), 11–12, 120–24; financial security in old age in US (1890–1950), 113–20, 141–42; health care in Sweden (1950–present), 124–25, 130; health care in US (1950–present), 125–32; health inequities of, 130–31, 133–34, 135, 139; industrialism and creation of retirement, 112–13; informal/family-member caregivers, 134, 140; long-term care, 131–32; medical expenses, 109; reform of Swedish system (1990–present), 138–41, 149; saving for retirement in US (1990–present), 141–44; sixty-five as normal retirement age, 78, 110–11, 113, 114; social capital and social integration, 133–38, 141; social determinants of health, 107–8, 111–12, 144; union pension plans, 115–16. *See also specific programs*

right, access to health care as, 7, 61
Rogers, Joel, 105
Roosevelt, Franklin, 52, 54, 58, 78, 95–100, 118–19, 127
Roosevelt, Theodore, 46, 79, 81, 85
Rotch, Thomas, 38–40, 64
Roussel, Théophile, 33
Roussel Law (1874), France, 32–33, 37, 63
RU-486, 58

Saint-Exupéry, Antoine de, *The Little Prince*, 28
Sanderson, Priscilla, x
scarlet fever, 37
Scharlach, Andrew, 138
Schieber, Sylvester, 142
school lunches, 50
Second Amendment, 153
Second World War. *See* World War II
Sellers, Christopher, 80
"seven-crown reform" in Sweden, 125
sewer socialism, 154
Sheppard, Morris, 51
Sheppard-Towner Act (1921), US, 50–54, 55, 58, 60, 63
silicosis, 89
Smith, Stephen, 33
social capital and social integration for the elderly, 133–38
social Catholicism, 43–45, 48
social Darwinism, 34
social democracies versus US, health care in, 1–27, 159–83; challenges faced by social democracies, 147; COVID-19 pandemic and, 1–5, 146; decommodification of health, 13, 61, 156; defined, 2–5; definition of social democracies, vi, 2; development of social democracy in Germany, 78; government leadership, role of, 14–16; health inequities and overall population health, 21–22; health outcomes as measure of, 5–6, *6*, 16–18, *17*, 148; healthism and,